Tips and Tricks in DERMATOLOGIC PRACTICE

Tips and Tricks in DERMATOLOGIC PRACTICE

Editors

Ranjan C Raval MD DVD
Professor
Department of Dermatology
CU Shah Medical College
Surendranagar, Gujarat, India

Krina B Patel MD DVD
Professor and Head
Department of Dermatology
GMERS Medical College and Hospital, Sola
Ahmedabad, Gujarat, India

Co-editor

Neetisha Agarwal MBBS DNB (Skin)
Consultant Dermatologist and Cosmetologist
Novum Cutis Clinic
Ahmedabad, Gujarat, India
Ex-Senior Resident
Department of Dermatology
Smt NHL Municipal Medical College
Ahmedabad, Gujarat, India

Foreword
PB Haribhakti

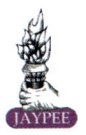

The Health Sciences Publisher
New Delhi | London | Panama

Jaypee Brothers Medical Publishers (P) Ltd

Headquarters
Jaypee Brothers Medical Publishers (P) Ltd
4838/24, Ansari Road, Daryaganj
New Delhi 110 002, India
Phone: +91-11-43574357
Fax: +91-11-43574314
Email: jaypee@jaypeebrothers.com

Overseas Offices

J.P. Medical Ltd
83, Victoria Street, London
SW1H 0HW (UK)
Phone: +44 20 3170 8910
Fax: +44 (0)20 3008 6180
Email: info@jpmedpub.com

Jaypee-Highlights Medical Publishers Inc
City of Knowledge, Bld. 235, 2nd Floor, Clayton
Panama City, Panama
Phone: +1 507-301-0496
Fax: +1 507-301-0499
Email: cservice@jphmedical.com

Jaypee Brothers Medical Publishers (P) Ltd
17/1-B, Babar Road, Block-B, Shaymali
Mohammadpur, Dhaka-1207, Bangladesh
Mobile: +08801912003485
Email: jaypeedhaka@gmail.com

Jaypee Brothers Medical Publishers (P) Ltd
Bhotahity, Kathmandu
Nepal
Phone: +977-9741283608
Email: kathmandu@jaypeebrothers.com

Website: www.jaypeebrothers.com
Website: www.jaypeedigital.com

© 2017, Jaypee Brothers Medical Publishers

The views and opinions expressed in this book are solely those of the original contributor(s)/author(s) and do not necessarily represent those of editor(s) of the book.

All rights reserved. No part of this publication may be reproduced, stored or transmitted in any form or by any means, electronic, mechanical, photocopying, recording or otherwise, without the prior permission in writing of the publishers.

All brand names and product names used in this book are trade names, service marks, trademarks or registered trademarks of their respective owners. The publisher is not associated with any product or vendor mentioned in this book.

Medical knowledge and practice change constantly. This book is designed to provide accurate, authoritative information about the subject matter in question. However, readers are advised to check the most current information available on procedures included and check information from the manufacturer of each product to be administered, to verify the recommended dose, formula, method and duration of administration, adverse effects and contraindications. It is the responsibility of the practitioner to take all appropriate safety precautions. Neither the publisher nor the author(s)/editor(s) assume any liability for any injury and/or damage to persons or property arising from or related to use of material in this book.

This book is sold on the understanding that the publisher is not engaged in providing professional medical services. If such advice or services are required, the services of a competent medical professional should be sought.

Every effort has been made where necessary to contact holders of copyright to obtain permission to reproduce copyright material. If any have been inadvertently overlooked, the publisher will be pleased to make the necessary arrangements at the first opportunity.

Inquiries for bulk sales may be solicited at: jaypee@jaypeebrothers.com

Tips and Tricks in Dermatologic Practice

First Edition: **2017**

ISBN 978-93-85891-60-1

Printed at: Sanat Printers

Dedicated to

*All our patients who gave us opportunity to learn and made us wiser.
We are thankful to all contributors for sharing their best work with us.*

Contributors

Aarti Shah MD DV&D
Consultant Dermatocosmetolgist
and Assistant Professor
Department of Dermatology
NHL Municipal Medical College
Ahmedabad, Gujarat, India

Ashish Jagati MD
Assistant Professor
Department of Dermatology
BJ Medical College
Ahmedabad, Gujarat, India

Asok Gangopadhyay
MD DVD FRCP
Professor and Head
Department of Dermatology
RKM Seva Pratishthan
Kolkata, West Bengal, India

BC Kamdar DV& D
Honorary Dermatologist with
Wockhardt Hospital
Rajkot, Gujarat, India
Managing Trustee
RB Kothari Polydiagnostic Centre
and Hospital
Founder Chief Editor
"Quarterderm".
Past President
IADVL, GSB 1987

Bela Shah MD
Professor and Head
Department of Dermatology
BJ Medical College
Ahmedabad, Gujarat, India

Bharat Shah MD
Senior Consultant Dermatologist
Ahmedabad, Gujarat, India
Ex-Professor and Head
Department of Dermatology
BJ Medical College
Ahmedabad, Gujarat, India

Bharati K Patel
Professor
PDU Medical College
Rajkot, Gujarat, India

Deep Joshipura MBBS MD
Clinical Research Fellow
Department of Dermatology
Tufts Medical Center
Boston, USA
Ex-Assistant Professor
Dermatology
Gujarat Adani Institute of Medical
Sciences, Bhuj, Gujarat, India

FE Billimoria MD
Professor and Head
Department of Dermatology
SBKS Medical Institute and
Research Center
Vadodara, Gujarat, India

Hasmukh J Shroff MD
Senior Consultant Dermatologist
Saifee Hospital
Mumbai, Maharashtra, India
Ex-Professor and Head
Department of Dermatology & STD
GMC & Sir JJ Group of Hospitals
Mumbai, Maharashtra, India

Hemangi R Jerajani
MD DVD FIAD
Professor and Head
Department of Dermatology
Venereology and Leprosy
MGM Medical College and
Hospital, Navi Mumbai
Maharashtra, India

JN Dave MD
Professor and Head
Department of Dermatology
CU Shah Medical College
Surendranagar, Gujarat, India

Keyur Shah DDV
HIV Consultant
Practicing Dermatologist
Ahmedabad, Gujarat, India

Kiran Godse MD FRCP
Professor
DY Patil School of Medicine
Navi Mumbai, Maharashtra, India

Kirti S Parmar MD
Associate Professor
BJ Medical College
Ahmedabad, Gujarat, India

Krina B Patel DV&D MD
Professor and Head
Department of Dermatology
GMERS Medical College
Sola
Ahmedabad, Gujarat, India

Monal Shah MD DVD
Consultant Dermatologist
Haribhakti Skin Clinic
Ahmedabad, Gujarat, India

Neela Patel DV&D MD
Professor and Head
AMC MET Medical College
Ahmedabad, Gujarat, India

Neela V Bhuptani MD
Professor and Head
PDU Medical College
Rajkot, Gujarat, India

Neetisha Agarwal DNB (Skin)
Consultant Dermatologist and
Cosmetologist
Novum Cutis Clinic
Ahmedabad, Gujarat, India

Nina Madnani MD DVD FISSVD
Consultant
PD Hinduja Hospital and Sir HN
Reliance Foundation Hospital
Mumbai, Maharashtra, India

PB Haribhakti
MD MRCPE (Dermatology) FRCPE
FAAD (USA) FIAMS
Senior Consultant Specialist in Skin,
Hair Disorders, Leprosy and STD
Haribhakti Skin Clinic
Ahmedabad, Gujarat, India

Palak Gandhi MD Dermatology
Consultant Dermatologist
Haribhakti Skin Clinic
Ahmedabad, Gujarat, India

Ranjan C Raval MD DVD
Professor
Department of Dermatology
CU Shah Medical College
Surendranagar, Gujarat, India

Rekha B Solanki MD
Professor
Department of Dermatology
Smt NHL Municipal Medical
College
Ahmedabad, Gujarat, India

Rita Vora MD
Professor and Head
Department of Dermatology
Pramukhswami Medical College
Karamsad, Gujarat, India

Saurabh Jindal MD DNB
Associate Professor
Department of Dermatology
Venereology and Leprosy
MGM Medical College and
Hospital
Navi Mumbai, Maharashtra, India

Sejal Thakkar MD DVD DCAH
Associate Professor
Department of Dermatology
GMERS Medical College
Gotri, Vadodara, Gujarat, India

Sharmila Patil MD
Professor and Head
DY Patil Medical College
Navi Mumbai, Maharashtra, India

Shaurya Rohatgi MD
Assistant Professor
Department of Dermatology
MGM Medical College and
Hospital
Navi Mumbai, Maharashtra, India

Shylaja Someshwar DVD DNB
Associate Professor
Department of Dermatology
Venereology and Leprosy
MGM Medical College and Hospital
Navi Mumbai, Maharashtra, India

Som J Lakhani MD
Assistant Professor
Department of Dermatology
SBKS Medical Institute and
Research Centre
Vadodara, Gujarat, India

Sudhir Pujara MD DVD DDV
Senior Consultant Dermatologist
Former Professor and Head
Department of Dermatology
Smt NHL Municipal Medical
College, and
Smt Shardaben Municipal
Hospital
Ahmedabad, Gujarat, India

Sujata Sengupta MD DCH
Associate Professor
Department of Dermatology
KPC Medical College
Kolkata, West Bengal, India

Suresh Joshipura
MD FRCP (Lond) PhD FAAD DVD
Consultant Dermatologist
Rajkot, Gujarat, India
Former Director of Research
HJ Doshi Medical Research
Foundation
Rajkot, Gujarat, India

YS Marfatia MD
Professor and Head
Department of Dermatology
Baroda Medical College
Vadodara, Gujarat, India

CONTRIBUTOR RESIDENT DOCTORS

Abhishek Pilani
Ipsa Pandya
Karam Vir Singh
Maitrey J Patel
Nidhi Livani
Nilofar Diwan
Vibhakar Vachharajani

Editorial

Science and in particular medical science is an ever expanding field with lots of research going on continuously. Research not only in laboratory but also in clinical settings in terms of day-to-day patient care enriches us in terms of experience we gain.

This innovative book is an endeavor to present the practical experiences of leading dermatology practitioners from India in the field of individual patient care. All the chapters from contributing authors are from their personal experiences in diagnosing and treating difficult patient or their own innovations in treating various skin conditions out of their own experience. You will find lots of tips from senior dermatologists to help you in day-to-day practice.

The book is a collection of some rare to difficult to treat cases as well as treatment options which may be beyond standard textbooks. This book is an attempt to make PG students and practitioners understand importance of even anecdotal cases and innovative treatment modalities. The book is in no particular order and one can read any chapter in random fashion as per their interest in subject.

We hope that you all will love to read this book and everyone will gain something out of it.

Ranjan C Raval
Krina B Patel
Neetisha Agarwal

Foreword

I have the good fortune to write a foreword for the book on *Tips and Tricks in Dermatologic Practice*.

It is always said that common things are very common but that does not imply that rare diseases can be forgotten. A good clinician is the one who is constantly reminded of something unusual in a case which he examines. The diagnosis of rare and uncommon conditions has a lot of implications in their management. The book gives insight into rare and unusual cases written by senior and experienced dermatologists. **Editorial Comments** at the end of every case is worth remembering.

The authors have done an uphill task of coordinating the clinical material available to them and putting them in a readable manner. I give my compliments to the authors and hope they continue to serve the Dermatology fraternity.

PB Haribhakti
MD MRCPE (Dermatology)
FRCPE FAAD (USA) FIAMS
Senior Consultant Specialist in Skin,
Hair Disorders, Leprosy & STD
Haribhakti Skin Clinic
Narayan Chambers, Nehrubridge Corner
Ashram Road, Amedabad, Gujarat, India

Preface

As all of us know that clinical dermatology is a vast field which includes common as well as rare diseases or common disease with rare presentation. Sometimes the diseases are recalcitrant to the evidence base guidelines or standard therapy so at this place experience comes into count.

In the world of clinical dermatology many diseases are there which can be diagnosed and managed by the experienced dermatologists by their knowledge and expertise which may not be according to the guidelines but the results are miraculous.

This book is an opportunity for all of us to gain from senior dermatologists who have not published their different but unique experiences which they are sharing with us. This may change our view to look at the disease in a different and exclusive way and also it will be of great help and guidance to the new budding dermatologists who may use these experiences as evidence in their future practice.

This book will share the experience and art of management of our senior and eminent dermatologists. This book will also include general tips and tricks in day-to-day clinical practice.

After all experience is the most valuable thing we can share with each other!

Ranjan C Raval
Krina B Patel
Neetisha Agarwal

Contents

1. **Photoexposed Papules and Plaques of Sarcoidosis: How We Treat** — 1
   Asok Gangopadhyay, Sujata Sengupta
   - Case No. 1 1
   - Case No. 2 3
   - Case No. 3 4

2. **Alopecia Totalis and Systemic Amyloidosis** — 7
   Aarti Shah

3. **Disseminated Histoplasmosis in a Patient of Acute Lymphocytic Leukemia: A Rare Case Report** — 9
   Bela Shah

4. **Langerhans Cell Histiocytosis** — 13
   Bela Shah, Ashish Jagati

5. **Eternal Student in Dermatology** — 18
   Bharat Shah

6. **Lupus Vulgaris** — 19
   Bharati K Patel

7. **Tips and Tricks in the Practice of Clinical Dermatology** — 21
   BC Kamdar

8. **Diffuse Cutaneous Leishmaniasis** — 26
   FE Bilimoria, Som J Lakhani, Karam Vir Singh, Maitreyi J Patel
   - Case No. 1 26
   Cutaneous T-Cell Lymphoma Mimicking Pemphigus 28
   - Case No. 2 28
   Rowell's Syndrome 30
   - Case No. 3 30

9. **Knowing Your Customer in Dermatology Practice** — 32
   Hasmukh J Shroff
   - The Customer is Always Right! 33

10. **Hypnosis in Dermatology** — 35
    JN Dave
    - Other Skin Conditions Where Hypnosis is Helpful 37

11. **Oil Melanosis** — 39
    JN Dave
    - Case No. 1 39
    Nail Pitting 40
    - Case No. 2 40
    Hair Loss 41
    - Case No. 3 41

12.	**Endurance and Patience** *Krina Bharat Patel*	**44**
13.	**Verruca Plana Treated with Oral Acitretin** *Kiran Godse* ■ Case No. 1 49 *Molluscum Contagiosum 50* ■ Case No. 2 50	**49**
14.	**Case Reports on Methotrexate Toxicity** *Kirti S Parmar*	**54**
15.	**Neglected Nevi: A Stitch in Time Saves Nine** *Kirti S Parmar* ■ Case No. 1 59 ■ Case No. 2 60	**59**
16.	**AIDS Cholangiopathy** *Keyur Shah, Neetisha Agarwal*	**63**
17.	**CD4 and Viral Load Discordance** *Keyur Shah, Neetisha Agarwal*	**68**
18.	**VZV Encephalitis with IRIS in PML** *Keyur Shah, Neetisha Agarwal*	**74**
19.	**Case Reports** *Keyur Shah, Neetisha Agarwal*	**78**
20.	**Trichofolliculoma Presenting as Verrucous Growth** *Neela Patel*	**83**
21.	**Acute Myeloid Leukemia** *Neela V Bhuptani*	**86**
22.	**Rare Case Reports** *Nina Madnani* ■ Case No. 1 88 ■ Case No. 2 89	**88**
23.	**Guidelines in Dermatology** *PB Haribhakti, Monal Shah, Palak Gandhi* *Orofacial Granulomatosis 92* ■ Case No. 1 92 *Epidermodysplasia Verruciformis 94* ■ Case No. 2 94	**91**
24.	**Leprosy Mimicking as Psoriasis** *Rita Vora, Abhishek Pilani, Nilofar Diwan, Nidhi Livani* ■ Case No. 1 96 ■ Case No. 2 98	**96**
25.	**Our Experience with Clinical Dermatology** *Ranjan C Raval, Neetisha Agarwal* ■ Case No. 1 102 ■ Case No. 2 103 ■ Case No. 3 104 ■ Case No. 4 104 ■ Case No. 5 105	**102**

26.	**Cutaneous Myiasis** Rekha B Solanki	**106**
27.	**Majocchi's Granuloma** Sharmila Patil	**107**

- Case No. 1   107

Resistant Tinea Corporis Infection   108

- Case No. 2   108

Eczematous Reaction to BCG Vaccination   110

- Case No. 3   110

28.	**Interesting Case Reports** Sudhir Pujara	**112**

- Case No. 1   112
- Case No. 2   112
- Case No. 3   113

29.	**Counselling and Peer Discussion: An Additional Intervention in Pemphigus Vulgaris!** Sejal Thakkar	**115**

- Case No. 1   115
- Case No. 2   116

30.	**An Interesting Case of Necrobiosis Lipoidica Diabeticorum and Trichotillomania: Tips and Tricks** Suresh Joshipura, Deep Joshipura, Vibhakar Vachharajani	**118**

- Case No. 1   118
- Case No. 2   119

31.	**Thorough Clinical Examination is the Key to Diagnosis** YS Marfatia, Ipsa Pandya	**122**
32.	**Diagnostic and Therapeutic Conundrums in a Case of Pemphigus Vulgaris** Shaurya Rohatgi, Hemangi R Jerajani, Saurabh Jindal, Shylaja Someshwar	**125**

Index   *131*

Chapter 1

Photoexposed Papules and Plaques of Sarcoidosis: How We Treat

Asok Gangopadhyay, Sujata Sengupta

CASE NO. 1

- **Age:** 63 years
- **Sex:** Female

Duration of the Disease

6 months

History

She complained of itchy skin lesions on her forehead, arms and upper back. She complained of photosensitivity in the lesions but no systemic symptoms.

Clinical Examination (General and Cutaneous)

General survey and systemic examinations were normal. Mildly erythematous papules and coalescing plaques were seen on the forehead, extensor aspects of the arms extending from the dorsum of the hands till the elbows and the upper back (Fig. 1). On the back, the coalescing plaques had infiltrated raised borders and shiny atrophic centers (Fig. 2). Mucous membranes, hair and nails were normal.

Differential Diagnosis

a. PMLE
b. Sarcoidosis.

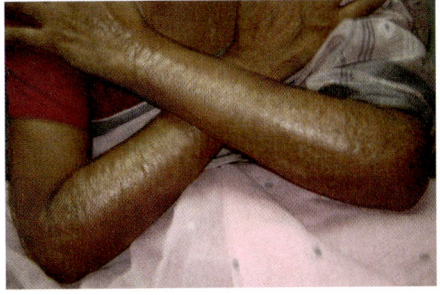

Fig. 1: Mildly erythematous papules and plaques on extensors of both forearms extending on dorsa of hands

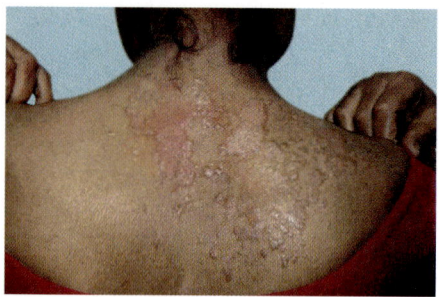

Fig. 2: Erythematous papules coalescing into plaques on photoexposed part of back

Investigations

Showed mild anemia, raised ESR (50mm) and negative Mantoux reaction, raised serum ACE (128U/l) and normal calcium.

Skin biopsy showed epithelioid granuloma with lymphocytes, occasional giant cells and no caseation

Final Diagnosis

Sarcoidosis involving photoexposed areas.

Management

We prescribed her a course of oral prednisolone and hydroxychloroquinesulphate 200mg twice daily, advised to apply sunscreen and topical fluticasone twice daily, but the lesions on her forearms did not show any encouraging results even after one and half months. We then gave her intralesional injections of triamcinolone (10mg/mL) on two occasions—1ml each time at multiple sites at the gap of 3 weeks and advised to apply tacrolimus ointment (0.1%) at night along with topical fluticasone once at daytime. We gradually tapered the dose of oral steroid but continued hydroxychloroquin. There was significant improvement in the lesions after one month (Figs 3 and 4).

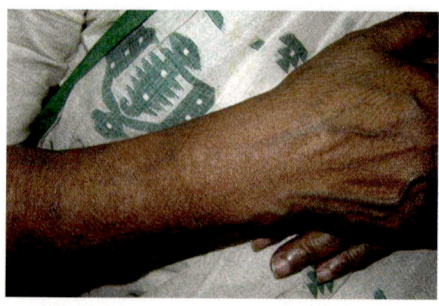

Fig. 3: Post-treatment photograph showing resolution of lesions

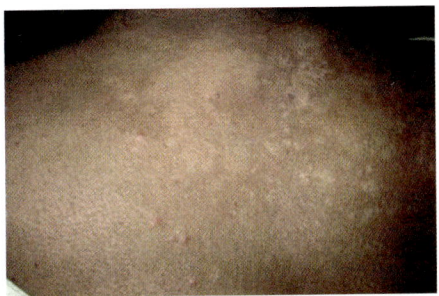

Fig. 4: Post-treatment partial resolution of lesions

CASE NO. 2

- **Age:** 42 years
- **Sex:** Female

Duration of the Disease

3 months

History

She presented with mildly-itchy skin lesions on both upper extremities for 3 months. There was redness and a burning sensation locally on sunexposure. Systemic symptoms were absent.

Clinical Examination (General and Cutaneous)

General and systemic examinations were normal. She had erythematous plaques and a few shiny papules confined to the extensor aspect of her arms and forearms (Fig. 5). No other skin lesions were seen elsewhere. Mucous membranes, hair and nails were normal.

Differential Diagnosis

a. Sarcoidosis
b. Polymorphous light eruption.

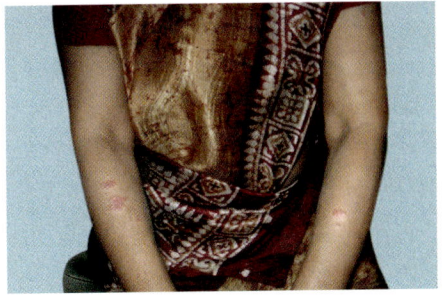

Fig. 5: Erythematous, shiny plaques on both forearms

Investigations

Raised ESR (60mm), negative Mantoux reaction, raised serum ACE (80U/l) and normal chest X-ray. Skin biopsy: Noncaseating granuloma, typical of sarcoidosis.

Final Diagnosis

Photosensitive sarcoidosis.

Management

We prescribed her oral hydroxy-choloroquine suphate and sunscreens. As topical application, fluticasone was given at daytime and tacrolimus (0.1%) at night. A follow-up of 4 months later showed clearing of the skin lesions (Fig. 6).

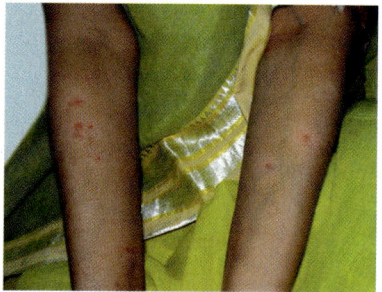

Fig. 6: Post-treatment resolution of lesions

CASE NO. 3

- **Age:** 35 years
- **Sex:** Male

Duration of the Disease

5 Months

History

He presented with asymptomatic raised skin lesions on upper chest for 5 months. The skin-coloured papules in the upper chest became itchy and red on sun exposure.

Clinical Examination (General and Cutaneous)

General and systemic examinations were normal. On the exposed parts of the chest, there were several skin-coloured papules and some annular plaques with raised borders and depressed atrophic centers (Fig. 7). Skin lesions were absent in the rest of the body and mucosae, hair and nails appeared unaffected.

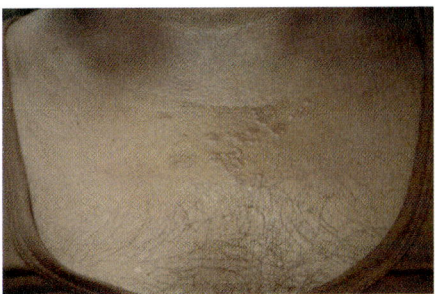

Fig. 7: Skin colored papules and annular plaques

Differential Diagnosis

a. Granuloma Annulare
b. Sarcoidosis.

Investigations

Raised ESR and negative Mantoux test. Skin biopsy revealed typical sarcoid granuloma.

Final Diagnosis

Photosensitive sarcoidosis.

Management

Sunscreen, oral hydroxychloroquine was advised along with topical fluticasone during the day and tacrolimus (0.1%) at night. Skin lesions subsided by 3 months (Fig. 8).

Tips for Managing Photosensitive Cutaneous Sarcoidosis

1. Sunscreens should be used in all cases of photoexposed lesions of sarcoidosis.
2. We advised once a day each application of fluticasone cream and tacrolimus ointment (0.1%) in these cases.
3. For resistant lesions, intralesional triamcinolone acetonide injections (10 mg/mL), are beneficial.

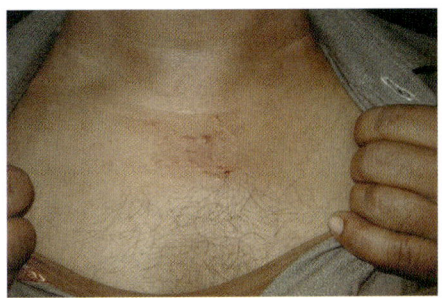

Fig. 8: Resolution of lesions after 3 months of treatment

> **Editorial Comments**
> - Some skin disease like photosensitive sarcoidosis can present as photodermatitis or actinic granuloma annulare
> - Photodermatitis is a common presentation and can turn out to be disease like sarcoidosis or Jessner's lymphoma or Lymphocytoma cutis on detailed examination and investigations.

Chapter 2

Alopecia Totalis and Systemic Amyloidosis

Aarti Shah

A 53-year-old female patient presented with alopecia totalis and loss of eyelashes since 2 years, oedema with asymptomatic papulonodular lesions on both lower limbs since 3 years and few hemorrhagic bullous lesions over both hands since 7–10 days. Facial edema and yellowish hue of face was seen and woody hard abdomen was palpated.

INVESTIGATIONS

She was anemic and had leucocytosis. The RFT showed severe proteinuria (4+). Urine examination showed presence of albumin (4+), few RBCs, pus cells. Serum A/G ratio was low. Hypothyroidism was also detected. Periorbital ecchymosis and macroglossia were absent. USG abdomen showed presence of multiple 1–2 cm sized lymphnodes in right inguinal region with subcutaneous edema in lower abdominal wall.

Serum protein electrophoresis showed albumin—45.6%, alpha 1–3.5%, alpha 2–23.1%, beta 1–13.3%, beta 2–4.7%, gamma 9.8%. No abnormal band was seen. Urine protein immune electrophoresis showed total protein—231.4, albumin 59.9, alpha 1–2.7, beta 37.4 and free kappa light chain (22.33). 24-hour urinary protein report showed reading of 4,357 (mg/day). ANA blot was negative. p-ANCA and c-ANCA were negative. Colour doppler showed no significant findings. S.HIV was negative.

Histopathological examination showed focal epidermal atrophy, hyperkeratosis and acanthosis in the epidermis. Upper dermis showed increased fibroblasts and collagen. Superficial perivascular and periappendageal lymphoplasmacytic inflammatory infiltrate and few periappendageal foreign body giant cells S/O *scleredema adultorum*.

Renal biopsy specimen showed basement membrane thickening and deposition of PAS negative material in mesangium (Congo red and Thio-T are positive). Tubular interstitial fibrosis and tubular atrophy with mild fibro-intimal thickening of vessels present. Immunofluorescence—C3: nonspecific mesangial staining, IgM-non specific mesangial staining, IgA and C1q, IgG—Negative. S/O renal amyloidosis.

TREATMENT

Patient was treated by oncologist with oral melphalan 10 mg daily in two divided doses and oral steroids but patient died of pleural effusion due to cardiac failure (? amyloid deposition) after 3 months of presentation at OPD.

DISCUSSION

The most common form of systemic amyloidosis is AL resulting from fibril formation by fragments of monoclonal antibody light chains resulting from plasma cell dyscrasia. The mean age of onset of primary amyloidosis is about 65 years and male preponderance is seen. Amyloidogenic immunoglobulin AL monoclonal proteins appear to be preferentially of gamma type, of lower molecular weight and lower isoelectric point. Fewer than 20% patients with AL have myeloma and 15–20% patients with myeloma have amyloidosis, the reason being production of amyloid fibrils on digestion of Bence Jones proteins. Abnormal light chain material is almost always present in serum or urine and can be demonstrated in tissue culture of bone marrow cells from affected patients. The organ tropism in AL amyloidosis may reflect germ line gene use and plasma cell burden.

CONCLUSION

We presented this case of primary systemic amyloidosis as a rare cause of alopecia totalis.

Our case was unique as it was associated with multiple myeloma and scleredema.

> **Editorial Comments**
> - Sometimes the common skin disease may reflect internal disorders proving skin to be mirror of body
> - In this unique case alopecia areata turned out to be the manifestation of multiple myeloma with primary systemic amyloidosis.

Chapter 3

Disseminated Histoplasmosis in a Patient of Acute Lymphocytic Leukemia: A Rare Case Report

Bela Shah

INTRODUCTION

Histoplasmosis also known as Darling's disease is a highly infectious mycosis but rare in India. It is usually caused by the dimorphic fungus, *Histoplasma capsulatum*. Skin lesions are more common with *H. duboisii* than with *H. capsulatum*. The disease spectrum varies from a mild respiratory infection to a lethal, disseminated form. The fungus is intracellular, parasitizing the reticuloendothelial system and involving the spleen, liver, kidney, central nervous system and other organs. Disseminated form is more common in the immune-compromised host. Here, we present a case of disseminated histoplasmosis in patient of acute lymphocytic leukemia (ALL).

Case Report

A 15-year-old female patient, studying in 10th standard, residing in Ahmedabad city of Gujarat, born of non-consanguineous marriage presented to our skin OPD with complaint of skin lesions since one month. Upon review, the patient was found to be undergoing treatment for ALL since past 2 years. She had history of recurrent platelet transfusions for the same. Along with that she was given allopurinol, vincristine, cyclophosphamide, 6-mercaptopurine, G-CSF, daunorubicin in various doses at the cancer institute of our hospital.

She gave history of multiple, discrete, nontender, papulo-nodular lesions all over body, predominantly over face and trunk since past one month. On taking detailed history, she was found to have associated complaint of productive cough and intermittent low-grade evening fever with weight loss and loss of appetite.

She had no history of Tuberculosis or other lung disease in her family.

Her physical examination revealed that she was conscious, emaciated and had fever with temperature of 102 degree Fahrenheit. Pallor was present. Her respiratory examination revealed a respiratory rate of 25 cycles/minute. Liver was 3 finger enlarged with splenomegaly. Her other vital signs were normal.

On cutaneous examination, she had multiple, discrete papulonodular lesions with umbilication all over the body. Few of the larger lesions showed crusting and scaling at the center of the nodule (Figs 1A and B).

On examination of reticuloendothelial system she was found to have generalized lymphadenopathy and hepatosplenomegaly.

A complete blood count revealed neutropenia and leucopenia. Hemoglobin levels were reduced to 10 mg/dl, total white blood cell count 2400 cells/mm^3 and platelet count 1 lac cells/mm^3. Her erythrocyte sedimentation rate was 22 mm/hour. Her renal and liver function tests were within normal limits. A rapid test for HIV was performed and was negative. Sputum tests for Gram staining and Ziehl–Nielsen staining were both found to be negative. Patient had multiple, hilar and apical, calcific densities present on chest roentgenogram at the time of diagnosis of her leukemia.

Biopsy of the skin was taken from a nodular lesion and sent for histopathological examination, which showed findings of epitheloid granuloma with fungal elements suggestive of histoplasmosis (Fig. 1C).

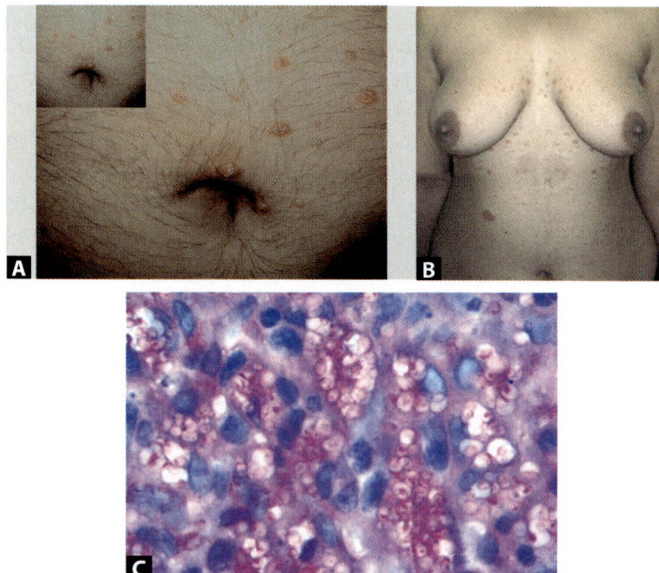

Figs 1A to C: (A and B) Multiple, discrete papulonodular lesions with umbilication all over the body with crusting and scaling at the center of the nodule; (C) Epithelioid granuloma with fungal elements suggestive of histoplasmosis (PAS Stain)

Bone marrow was sent for culture at 25° and 37°C for fungal growth. At 25°C, characteristic tuberculate macroconidia developed further supporting our clinical impression of disseminated histoplasmosis.

Because of resource limitations at our hospital, no further tests could be performed.

TREATMENT

The patient was given Injection Amphotericin B 65 mg in 500 ml of 5% dextrose over 4 hours for one month at the cancer institute along with chemotherapeutic drugs she was already on for the ALL.

Then she was shifted to T. Itraconazole 200 mg twice daily along with 6-mercaptopurine 50mg at night and T. methotrexate 15mg once per week.

DISCUSSION

In this report, we describe the case of a 15-year-old immune compromised female patient, a known case of ALL who presented to our hospital with multiple papulonodular skin lesions associated with fever and weight loss. This case illustrates that a rare clinical suspicion when supported with significant history, detailed examination and appropriate investigations helps in coming to a rare diagnosis of disseminated histoplasmosis which guides proper management of the patient.

The endemic fungi which are primarily human pathogens and whose major portal of entry is the respiratory tract include *H. capsulatum, Blastomyces dermatitidis* and *Coccidioides immitis*. Histoplasmosis has been shown to be a benign, self-limiting infection in most cases, but fatal cases have also been reported. The main route of acquisition could be airborne contamination from the soil and rarely, direct inoculation.

Histoplasma capsulatum exists as a saprophyte in nature, and has often been isolated from soil, particularly when contaminated with chicken feathers or droppings. Other birds, such as starlings, and bats have also been implicated in the establishment of saprophytic reservoirs of infection. The fungus has been demonstrated in the soil of caves inhabited by bats, and in endemic areas histoplasmosis is recognized as a hazard to cave explorers.

Histoplasma capsulatum var. capsulatum has been isolated from the organs and faeces of house dwellings bats in Panama. Its spores are infectious not only to humans, but also to small animals such as dogs, cats and rats. The disease is not transmitted from human to human or from animal to human, but by the inhalation of air-borne conidia. Epidemics have occurred from time to time among people exposed to spore charged atmospheres when exploring caves or cleaning out sites rich in the excrement of birds. Infection may follow introduction of spores through skin and mucous membranes, as in laboratory workers. Lymphoma appears to favor the development of the infection. In addition, histoplasmosis is an important complicating infection in patients with AIDS.

Culture remains the gold standard for the diagnosis of histoplasmosis, but it requires a lengthy incubation period (two to four weeks). Fungal staining produces quicker results than culture but is less sensitive.

The choice of therapy for histoplasmosis has become considerably wider in recent years. For many disseminated or localized forms of the disease, oral itraconazole is highly effective but has a high relapse rate, with a one-year relapse rate of 95.3% having been reported. Treatment with fluconazole 200–400 mg daily appears to be even less effective. An alternative in severe cases is amphotericin B. Successful treatment with voriconazole and posaconazole have also been described. Mortality associated with severe histoplasmosis without treatment is 80% but can be reduced to < 25% with antifungal therapy.

CONCLUSION

Although more common in immunecompromised patients, disseminated histoplasmosis should be considered in the differential diagnosis of patients with risk factors like leukemia who are on chemotherapeutic drugs making them susceptible to infections. Early diagnosis and treatment are important to improve outcomes.

CONSENT

Written informed consent was obtained from the patient's parents to publish this case report and any accompanying images.

Editorial Comments

Papulonodular lesions are common presentation of skin disease and usually are infective and inflammatory in origin but in immunocompromised patients rare disease like histoplasmosis should be thought of. Thorough systemic examination and related investigations should be done to rule out any systemic involvement.

Chapter 4

Langerhans Cell Histiocytosis

Bela Shah, Ashish Jagati

CASE NO. 1

- **Age:** 4 years
- **Sex:** Male

Duration of the Disease

2 years

History

Child was relatively asymptomatic 3 years back, when he developed reddish flat-topped lesions which started on the upper back and gradually progressed to involve the entire trunk that subsequently healed leaving post-inflammatory depigmentation. He was treated as miliaria, seborrheic dermatitis and miliary tuberculosis by various physicians without any relief.

History of recurrent fever, chronic cough, polyurea and polydipsia were present.

Birth history was insignificant. No relevant family or personal history were there.

On Cutaneous Examination

- Multiple grouped, hypopigmented, scaly, 0.5-1cm sized macules interspersed with few erythematous papular lesions were present over the forehead, neck and trunk.
- Greasy scales present on an erythematous base over scalp, behind the ears (Figs 1 and 2).

On Palpation

- Multiple, irregular depressions were felt over the skull.
- Generalised Lymphadenopathy was present
- Hepatosplenomegaly were present.

On Ocular Examination

Exophthalmos was present.

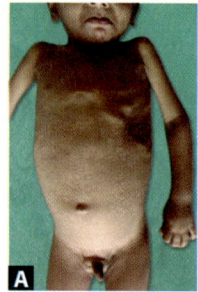

Fig. 1: Grouped, hypopigmented, scaly, 0.5-1 cm, macules interspersed with few erythematous papular lesions present over the forehead, neck and trunk

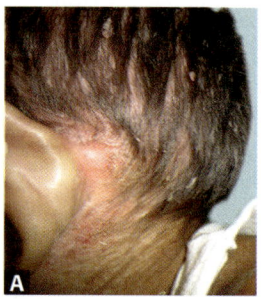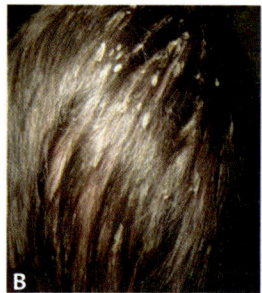

Fig. 2: Greasy scales present on an erythematous base

Investigations

- Microcytic, hypochromic anemia, thrombocytopenia.
- Total WBC count: WNL
- Blood urea nitrogen, blood sugar, serum electrolytes, etc. were within normal limits
- Urine specific gravity was low (1003) and daily urine output was about 6–7 liters
- Mantoux test, HIV: Negative
- Sputum AFB: Negative
- Cervical lymph node biopsy revealed nonspecific changes
- USG abdomen: Liver and spleen enlarged multiple hypoechoic lesions S/O splenic infiltration.
- X-ray skull showed punched out lesions (Fig. 3)
- X-ray chest showed multiple infiltrates in bilateral lungs (Fig. 4)
- CT scan showed compression of pituitary gland (Fig. 5).

Skin Biopsy

Histopathology: Skin biopsy showed lichenoid infiltrate of histiocytic cell in the upper dermis. These cells have pink cytoplasm and lobulated nuclei. There are few lymphocytes, eosinophils present below the histiocytic infiltrate (Fig. 6).

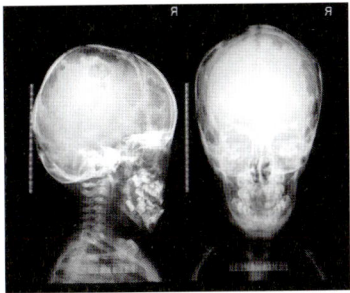
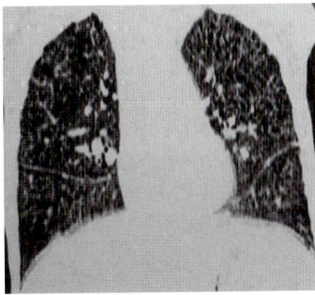

Fig. 3: Multiple geographic, punched-out lytic lesions in the skull, involving the parietal, temporal and frontal bones were seen

Fig. 4: Multiple ill-defined, variable size, bizzare shaped, cystic lesions distributed all over the lungs bilaterally

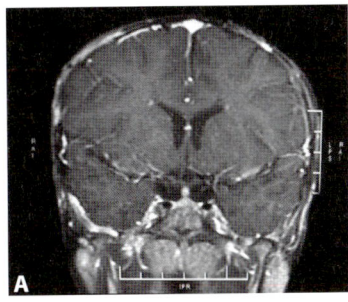
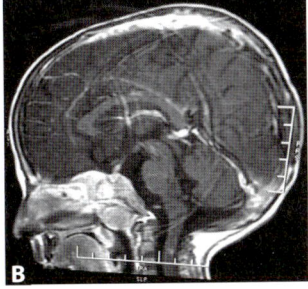

Fig. 5: Compression of pituitary gland at the level of sella turcica

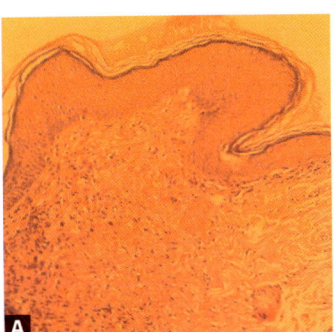
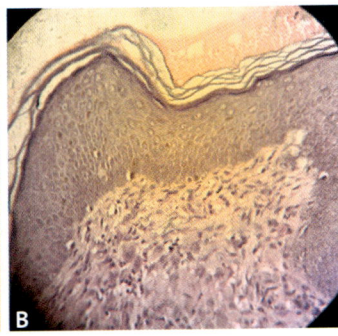

Fig. 6: Lichenoid infiltrate of histiocytes in upper dermis

On immunohistochemistry: The cells showed S-100, langerin and CD1a positivity.

Differential Diagnosis

a. Seborrheic dermatitis
b. Diaper dermatitis
c. Langerhans cell histiocytosis
d. Multiple myeloma (for bony lytic lesion)
e. Leukemia.

Final Diagnosis
Langerhans cell histiocytosis.

Management
Vinblastine 0.2 mg/kg weekly along with prednisone 2mg/kg/day (under the supervision of oncophysician). Patient was followed up and his general as well as cutaneous condition was improving.

DISCUSSION

Langerhans cell histiocytosis (LCH) is a clonal proliferative disease of Langerhans cells that expresses an immunophenotype positive for S100, CD1a and Langerin (CD207), and which contain cytoplasmic Birbeck granules.

Langerhans represents a disease spectrum with four prominent but overlapping syndromes:
1. Letterer–Siwe disease
2. Hand–Schüller–Christian disease
3. Eosinophilic granuloma
4. Congenital self-healing reticulohistiocytosis (Hashimoto–Pritzker disease).

Prevelance
4–5.4 per million population.
- **Age:** 2–6 years
- **Pathogenesis:** BRAFV600E mutation.

Skin Lesion
Lytic bone lesion, diabetes insipidus, and exophthalmos. Lung, liver, lymph nodes, spleen.

Recurrent Infection
Increased incidence of solid tumors and leukemia has been noted in patients previously treated for LCH.

Treatment
Chemotherapy—Oral and parentral steroids, vinablastine, etposide vemurafenib and dabrafenib for braf mutation.

Radiotherapy
Surgery: Bone curettage.
Mortality rate with multisystem disease: 35–55%.

PEARLS

Langerhans cell histiocytosis is the commonest of the histiocytic disorders. Owing to the relative rarity of the condition, it remains a disease in which the diagnosis is often delayed or missed.

Possibility of the diagnosis should always be entertained by the clinician and performing thorough systemic examination wherever feasible assumes special significance. Apart from clinical examination, proper evaluation of the hematologic, pulmonary, hepatosplenic, renal and skeletal systems to determine the extent of disease holds utmost importance. Further evaluation of CNS and bone marrow may be required. Patient should be referred to the Hematologist, oncologist and Pediatrician. Establishing early diagnosis after clinic-pathological corelation, early treatment initiation helps prevent disease related permanent consequences such as diabetes insipidus, endocrinopathies, orthopedic problems, hearing impairment, liver and lung failure and CNS disease.

Suggested Readings

1. Badalian-Very G, Vergilio J, Degar BA, et al. Recurrent BRAF mutations in Langerhans cell histiocytosis. Blood. 2010;116: 1919-23.
2. Chu A, D'Angio GJ, Favara BE, et al. Histiocytosis syndromes in children. Lancet. 1987;2:41-2.
3. Gadner G, Grois N, Arico M, et al. A randomized trial of treatment for multisystem Langerhans' cell histiocytosis. J Pediatr. 2001;138:728-34.
4. Willman CL, Busque L, Griffith BB, et al. Langerhans'-cell histiocytosis (histiocytosis X)—a clonal proliferative disease. N Engl J Med. 1994;331:154-60.

Chapter 5

Eternal Student in Dermatology

Bharat Shah

When I was a student in dermatology, there was one reference book which was called Sutton and Sutton. Venereology was not stressed much but now it is under the heading of sexually transmitted diseases (STD). Sexually transmitted diseases is being defined as prophylaxis and contraception in vogue.

For a student now, several textbooks, reference books and monograms are available. As dermatology is divided into 3 branches, dermatology venereology and leprology, there is lots and lots to read for students and even at times students fall short of time to learn.

Now new avenues will open up under the heading of outer space dermatology. Environmental pollution, chemicals, cosmetics also play a great role in the subject of dermatology. As age advances, newer chemicals, newer drugs and newer mechanical devices are in the arms of treatment.

With knowledge of STD and use of protective contraceptives, STD is in decline.

Genital problems are on an increase due to use and abuse of antibiotics, steroids and admixture of both. The problem of balanoposthitis, vaginitis and cervicitis is on an increase.

Drugs, chemicals, medicines, food preservatives, additives, colors, essences, combination of all of these, cold and hard drinks, tonics and purgatives are regularly being flooded in the market, which could be a source of allergen or irritant.

As a student I was taught that patients don't die of skin diseases and don't get better for eternity. One of my teachers quote this into a simple axiom that "some diseases are treated internally, some diseases externally but skin diseases are treated eternally"

Long live dermatology!!!

> **Editorial Comments**
> - Everyone out here in this world is a student. Learning never stops
> - We are grateful to the great teachers, seniors, colleagues and juniors who gave this opportunity to us.

Chapter 6

Lupus Vulgaris

Bharati K Patel

CASE NO. 1

- **Age:** 17 years
- **Sex:** Male

Duration

4 Years

History

An Orthopedic surgeon asked us on phone to give advice regarding treatment of their patient having biopsy finding s/o fungal element after scrapping of material from recurrent pus discharging lesion on left hand since 4 years. HP report was suggestive of Mycetoma showing filamentous structure in PAS stain.

We asked them to refer the patient to skin OPD for clinical examination as there can not be filamentous structure in PAS stain if it is mycetoma. There was H/O injury over left hand by stone before 4 years following he developed recurrent pus discharging lesion on left hand for which he had undergone many surgical procedures. There was H/O pulmonary TB in mother.

Clinical Findings

Multiple discharging sinuses were present with hyperpigmentation and hypertrophy of thenar eminence. Single ulcer was present over dorsa of left hand. Single round plaque with central atrophic scarring and hypopigmentation was noted over left lower forearm. Left axillary lymph node was palpable. Biopsy was taken from the plaque.

Investigations

CBC showed hypochromic microcytic anaemia

Histopathological finding was suggestive of lupus vulgaris, X-ray left arm: Periosteal reaction suggestive of osteomyelitis.

Final Diagnosis

Lupus vulgaris.

Patient responded well to AKT and lesions got healed completely.

Treatment

AKT Cat–I for 6 months.

> ### *Tips*
> - In any patient, treatment advice should not be given on telephone even to a doctor. Detailed history and thorough clinical examination of patient should always be done.

Chapter 7

Tips and Tricks in the Practice of Clinical Dermatology

BC Kamdar

INTRODUCTION

The one who thought of editing a book of this magnitude deserves compliments. Half-centurian dermatologist like me will think:

- Will it be appropiate in the present scenario to publish such an epic where cosmetology and dermatosurgery has overtaken the clinical dermatology?
- Whether budding dermatologists will be interested in going through this book!
- Whether upcoming dermatologists appreciate this colossal effort!
- Whether this book recreate the interest of present-day dermatologists towards clinical aspect of the vast field of dermatology!

However, in the larger context, this is going to be very much helpful in applying nonevidenced, evidenced and practical approach to the problem which is not scientifically understood.

PRESENT SCENARIO

Cosmetic and surgical dermatology have overtaken the clinical dermatology. Interest of dermatologists has shifted from clinical dermatology to cosmetic, surgical and procedural dermatology because it is more lucrative. Priorities of patients are also changed. Bulk of skin-blemishes' people seek advice of dermatologist. In the past, patients with acne, skin blemishes, tricholysis, male and female pattern baldness, premature greying, melasma-chloasma, tinea versicolor or hypertrichosis were hardly seeking advice of dermatologist. These days, this has become an outstanding priority.

ALL-THE-SAME

Old wine has always been better.

History

Taking a detailed relevent and irrelevent history is always highly rewarding.

Examples:
- A patient of chronic urticaria with dermatographism was treated with only tab. Liv-52 ds 1 BD for 6 mths with absolute cure because patient gave history of repeated attacks of hepatitis in the past.
- A patient of urticaria with angioneuritic edema repeatedly occuring in the same season, was finally relieved on avoiding flowering season of the neem tree in her compound.
- A patient of contact allergic dermatitis of hands was relieved on avoiding mixing of tea leaves in which he used to indulge occasionally.

There are many such examples. It proves beyond doubt that detailed history taking has to be an essential aspect of our approach to the final diagnosis.

Clinical Examination

Detailed and thorough examination of the patient from tip of the hair to the tip of the toe, including genitals is also equally rewarding.
- Diabetes mellitus is, times without number, first diagnosed by a dermatologist on examining prepuce.
- Scabies, lichen planus, psoraisis and many other diseases of skin can be diagnosed by regional examination.
- Examination of buccal cavity can throw light in arriving at correct diagnosis.
- Examination of the very first lesion to appear alongwith the last lesion to appear may prove to be diagnostic.
- Scrapping of every papulosquamous lesion should be a routine practice. It is capable of changing your diagnosis.
- You will need minimum number of investigations, minimum number of drugs as well as your patient will need shortest time to recover if you have taken detailed history and examined him/her thoroughly from tip of the hair to the tip of the toe.
- Common skin diseases form 90% of our practice whereas only 10% of uncommon skin diseases, account for our practice.
- Area of appearance of first lesion is capable of guiding us to a correct diagnosis.

Record Keeping

It was difficult to maintain records half a century back when I had started my practice. With the introduction of computers, it is much easier now. Serial photography and many examining devices with digital application are now available to dermatologist which makes record-keeping much better. This will help you in many ways.

1. Medicolegal
2. Saves time on follow-up visits.
3. Note of drug, food or other hypersensivity will help you to avoid mistakes.

Examples:
1. Way back in 1984, I was called upon to see a patient in a town some 60 kms. away, by a senior family physician. On casual inquiry, I was told that I had seen the same patient some 15 years back. While visiting the patient, I carried my old record of the same patient with me. Patient had severe generalised rash with intractable pruritus, erythema, fever, few lesions resembling fungus infection, few appeared bacterial infection. Family physician who had acompanied me told me that patient was receiving gresiofulvin, tetracycline, antihistamine, antipyretic and topically antifungal cream. From my record, I showed to the family physician that he himself had referred this patient to me for allergic reaction to tetracycline. On discontinuing tetracycline, everything went well.
2. A patient with severe and acute eczematoid perianal dermatitis visited my clinic. He had earlier come to me for herpes zoster. He was given xylocaine ointment for loal application to which, he had reacted badly. On enquiry, patient had piles and he was applying some ointment which was containing xylocaine which had resulted into acute perianal eczema. He improved only after discontuing pile's ointment.

Occupation

This is one of the most important area which we should unearth because these days number of industries use number of chemicals, farmers are using pesticides, fertilisers and preservatives; housewives are using detergents and other number of chemicals. On suspicion of occupational dermatitis, detailed history of indulgence in any such material will help in curing the patient.

Few Unusual Responses

- A patient of severe leprotic neuritis, responded only to tab. ancolan (an antihistaminic). Why and how? GOK. (god only knows). No other patient thereafter responded to this therapy.

- A patient of severely pruritic tinea cruris, responded to a single tablet of mexaform. Why and how? GOK.
- A case of recurrent psoriasis with erythematous base responded only to oral broad-spectrum antoibiotics for three weeks. Why and how? GOK.
- A case of psoriasis who consumed tab doxycycline daily for 2 ½ years without consulting the doctor, was relieved of psoriasis for 25 years.
- A patient of scleroderma with Reynaud's phenomenon, remained symptom-free for 3 years with tab complamina retard 1 OD, tab trental 400mg. 1 OD and tab deflazacort 6mg on alternate days.
- A patient of severely pruritic rash with chloroquin, resulting into hyperkeratosis and hyperpogmentation for number of years, was temporarily completely relieved with disappearence of hyperkeratosis and hyperpigmentation on receiving inj garamycin for five days to prevent infection after operation of cataract.
- A nonhealing ulcer on sole of foot of leprotic origin healed complelely with oral ofloxacin 200 mg daily for 6 mths.
- Dressing with mupirocin + metronidazple gel + placentrax gel has helped many patients with chronic nonhealing ulcer of static origin.
- Occlusive dressings with appropiate topicals on palms and soles are extremely gratifying.
- Tight-fitting dress with application of emolient ointment is helpful in senile pruritus.
- Lichen planus and psoriasis can reapppear even after 25 years.
- Some people never develop fungus infection. It seems to have genetic predesposition.
- Tab dapsone 100mg daily has helped in controlling lichen planus, vesiculobullous eruptions of unknown origin besides DH.
- Cyclophosphamide 50 mg. BD has helped similarly in controlling vesiculobullous, severely pruritic lesions of unknown origin.
- One should be very caucious in using clobetasone propionate. Its miraculous effect tends the patient to use it for a long time resulting into severe atrophy and hypopigmentation. Unfortunately, it is an OTC product. As in foreign countries, no one except dermatologist should be allowed to prescribe this product in India also. Chemist should be forced to keep the record of the sale of this product by the government.

Counseling

Its importance is known to every dermatologist. As skin disease is visible to the patient, the embarrasment is tremendous to cause psychological problems which should settled by counselling.

Method of Local Application

It is an important aspect of treatment. Failure to explain the method of application to the patient can result into failure to get desired results.

- From periphery to centre.
- Minimum amount
- Patient should be demonstrated the application of elastic bandage, corn-tape, chemically cauterising materials, occlusive dressings, shampoos, scalp applications, sprays, etc.

Our failure should not be because of faulty method of application.

Verdict and Message

Please spend half an hour with the patient on his/her visit, record the history, positive clinical findings and the line of treatment. This will curtail the time to a great extent on subsequent visit. Proper guidance for consuming medicine and local application alongwith counseling will yield better, faster and positive results. Patient's satisfaction and our gratification will be pleasant and heartwarming.

> **Editorial** Comments
> - Wow! No one but experienced, senior physician can guide us like this.
> - We all know but shall practice more.

Chapter 8

Diffuse Cutaneous Leishmaniasis

FE Bilimoria, Som J Lakhani, Karam Vir Singh, Maitreyi J Patel

CASE NO. 1

- **Age:** 40 years
- **Sex:** Male

Duration of the Disease

2 Years

History

History of fatigue, recurrent gastroenteritis and remarkable weight loss, since 6 months.

History of papulonodular lesions on face, trunk and extremities, involvement of oral and nasal mucosa and hoarseness of voice.

Sexual history positive for multiple unprotected extramarital sexual contacts.

No previous treatment taken.

Clinical Examination Revealed

a. Multiple, bilateral and asymptomatic papulonodular lesions on face, trunk and extremities (Figs 1A and B).
b. Infiltrations of oral and nasal mucosa with involvement of tongue, soft palate and posterior pharyngeal wall.

Differential Diagnosis

a. Disseminated cutaneous leishmaniasis
b. Lepromatous leprosy
c. Neurofibromatosis
d. Histoplasmosis
e. Cryptococcosis.

Investigations

a. Complete blood count—Normal
b. Serum HIV (by ELISA and Western blot)—Positive
c. CD4 count—95/cu mm
d. Giemsa Stain (of scraped material from lesions)—presence of 2–3 microns blue leishman bodies (Fig. 2A)

e. Skin biopsy—massive dermal invasion of lymphocytes and histiocytes with round cytoplasmic microgranules of 1–2 microns diameter (Fig. 2B).

Final Diagnosis

Diffuse cutaneous leishmaniasis

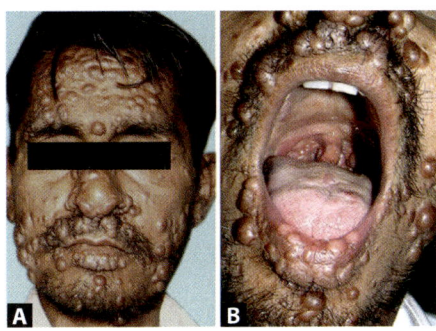

Figs 1A and B: (A) Photograph showing multiple papulonodular lesions. (B) Infiltration of oral mucosa and tongue

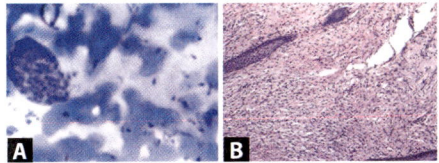

Figs 2A and B: Photographs showing (A) leishman bodies, (B) lympho-histiocytic infiltration with round cytoplasmic microgranules

Management

a. The patient was referred to ART centre and Antiretroviral therapy was started in the form of zidovudine, lamivudine and efavirenz.
b. Due to nonavailability of miltefosine the patient was put on combination therapy of ketoconazole 200mg twice daily and rifampicin 600mg once daily.

Tips and Comments

- This patient had an atypical and severe clinical presentation of cutaneous leishmaniasis in terms of number (>200), sites and types of lesions (papulonodular). Mucosal lesions in cutaneous leishmaniasis in an HIV patient should not be considered as mucocutaneous leishmaniasis (MCL) because parasites commonly disseminate and involve nasal and oral mucosa of body.
- Coinfection may amplify the immune defect against both leishmaniasis and HIV and increase disease severity and morbidity.
- Our patient responded very well to anti retroviral therapy and the lesions started subsiding as soon as ART was started. Ketoconazole may be a useful alternative to miltefosine and sodium stibogluconate, due to expense and nonavailability of these drugs.

We report this case because of:
a. Dual infection—Cutaneous leishmaniasis and HIV and
b. The presentation of diffuse cutaneous leishmaniasis masquerading as lepromatous leprosy.

> **Editorial Comments**
> - Leshmaniasis may sometimes mimic leprosy and only thorough clinical examination, smear and histopathology examination can confirm diagnosis and rule out other differential diagnosis.

Cutaneous T-Cell Lymphoma Mimicking Pemphigus

CASE NO. 2
- **Age:** 16 year
- **Sex:** Female

Duration of the Disease
6 Months

History
Multiple mildly pruritic skin lesions on the abdomen, back, thigh and limbs, since last 6 months.

No history of oral involvement, no other constitutional symptoms.

Patient was treated by private doctor and was given topical corticosteroids and antihistamines.

Clinical Examination (Figs 3A and B)
a. Multiple mildly pruritic papulovesicular lesions with crusting and scaling on the abdomen, back, thigh and limbs.
b. Patient later developed necrotising ulcers on the medial aspect of right thigh and on left lumbar region.

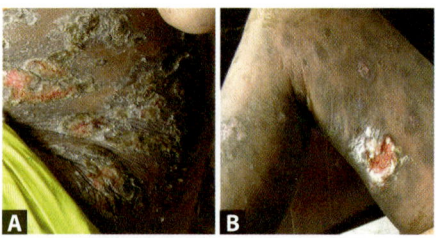

Figs 3A and B: (A) Showing multiple papulovesicular lesions with scaling and crusting over lower abdomen and (B) Showing single punched out ulcer over thigh

c. General examination revealed bilateral nontender inguinal lymphadenopathy.

Differential Diagnosis
a. Pemphigus vulgaris
b. Leukocytoclastic vasculitis
c. Cutaneous T-cell lymphoma.

Investigations
a. Routine investigations within normal limits.
b. Histopathological examination reveled epidermotrophism with intraepidermal Pautrier microabcesses containing atypical lymphocytes. Dermis showed marked lymphocytic infiltration (Fig. 4).
c. Histochemical markers positive for CD3, CD4, CD8 and negative for CD19, CD20 and CD30.

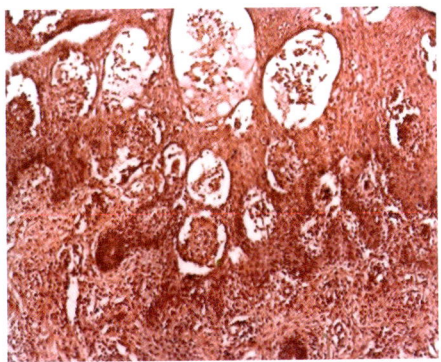

Fig. 4: Histopathological examination showing epidermotrophism with intraepidermal Pautrier microabcesses containing atypical lymphocytes

Final Diagnosis
Cutaneous T-cell lymphoma mimicking pemphigus.

Management
Treated with CHOP (cyclophosphamide 750mg, doxorubicin 60mg, vincristine 2mg) on day 1 and tablet prednisolone 80mg for 5 consecutive days. Five such cycles were given at an interval of 21 days.

Tips and Comments
- In any patient presenting with papulovesicular lesions not responding to corticosteroids and immunosuppresents a differential diagnosis of cutaneous T-cell lymphoma should be kept in mind.
- Repeated Biopsies are essential to come to the right diagnosis.
- A broad outlook and knowledge of the subject is essential for diagnosing such atypical cases.

Editorial Comments

- Strong suspicion for atypical cases like mentioned by the author should be kept in mind when presenting with common skin disease presentation
- Final diagnosis is made by biopsy.

Rowell's Syndrome

CASE NO. 3

- **Age:** 40 years
- **Sex:** Female

Duration of the Disease

3 Months

History

History of fever, joint pain, dryness in oral cavity since last 3 months.

History of skin lesions over face, back, palms and soles since last 2 months.

Photosensitivity since last 1 month.

History of Raynaud's phenomenon present since 1 month.

Clinical Examination (Figs 5A and B)

a. Erythematous atrophic plaques with adherent scales over both cheeks.
b. Target lesions over face, back, palms and soles.
c. Erosions present over hard palate and over buccal mucosa.

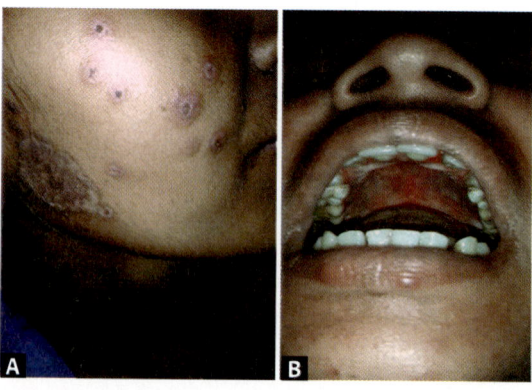

Figs 5A and B: Photographs showing (A) Erythematous atrophic plaques with adherent scales. (B) Erosions present over hard palate and over buccal mucosa

Differential Diagnosis
Subacute Cutaneous Lupus Erythematosus with Erythema Multiforme.

Investigations
a. Hb 8.9 mg%
b. Total count was within normal limits.
c. SGOT—103 IU/L (raised)
d. 24 hour urine protein—200mg (raised)
e. RA factor (+)
f. ANA (+++), Anti Sm- RNP (+), Anti Ro (+++), Anti La (+++)

Final Diagnosis
SCLE with EM (Rowell's Syndrome).

Management
Injectable Dexamethasone 1cc, once daily for 5 days, followed by TB. Prednisolone 30mg once daily, which was gradually tapered off, oral hydroxychloroquine 200mg twice daily and supportive treatment with healing of skin lesions and oral ulcers.

> ### Tips and Comments
> - Rowell's syndrome is a distinctive condition of cutaneous LE with lesions resembling EM on the face, neck, chest, hands and mouth.
> - In all patients with erythema multiforme it is prudent to look for associated connective tissue disorder.

Chapter 9

Knowing Your Customer in Dermatology Practice

Hasmukh J Shroff

Be it in business or profession, the importance of knowing your customer (KYC) well is vital to achieve good result. In my forty five years of dermatology practice I have learnt many lessons while dealing with patients and am still learning. It is a fascinating journey of realizing human mind.

While there are excellent sources for science of dermatology better than me I have few submissions on its art.

In any clinical practice doctor–patient relationship has two major objectives for the doctor, it is arriving at a diagnosis and delivering effective treatment, for the patient, it is to get relief early and cure ultimately.

Doctor endeavours to achieve his goal and patient has his own expectations.

What is it that You Would Like to Know About Your Patient?

There are **all kinds of patients**—poor and rich, literate and illiterate, regular and irregular, meticulous or casual, complying and noncomplying and so on. Some are internet savvy, some want to test your skill, while some are bargaining type. Approach of handling each patient has to be different. We know—'one size does not fit all!' Here it is the **skill and experience of treating physician** that makes all the difference in proper evaluation. This, aspect can determine if you can win the confidence of the patient or otherwise antagonize him/her.

Most important thing in clinical practice which my late father (also a dermatologist) taught me is to **put one's own self in patient's position** and then prescribe the treatment or advice accordingly. One has to be honest to the patient so that unnecessary expenses of investigations, procedure or drugs are avoided.

Often, but not always, it is possible to judge the patient from your long-standing experience as to where he could be hailing from, his ethnicity, mother tongue, affordability, etc. Based on this judgement your communication with the patient is facilitated. This way you could test yourself and even pleasantly surprise the patient. It helps to **build confidence and rapport with the patient.**

Lending ears to the patient and hearing him without interruptions yield quality information. Make the patient feel that you have enough time for him and are really involved in his problem. Never let the patient not feel that you have dealt with him in hurry. Besides, make the whole ambience lively, do not have serious face that can worry patient. In fact it is a good idea to crack a joke or two; yes in chamber practice and not ER.

Brief clinical notes on the prescription paper are helpful during subsequent follow-up. Revealing your care and concern about the patient by a phone call or other means go a long way in creating rapport. The silent message that must reach every patient is "I listen; I care".

We have to treat patient as whole not limiting to his dermatological problem only but attending also to his associated disease/conditions. Before discarding any drug for its inefficacy assess the reason. Although prompt symptomatic relief is important let the prescription be minimal and not a drug for each trivial complaint.

There are times when one is not able to make any diagnosis. What do you do in such a case? Depending on the type of patient you have and knowing his nature either you can inform him or buy time to refer books/journal, internet search, etc or discuss with senior colleagues for guidance. In any case let patient do not know of your confused state to arrive at a diagnosis.

Three things that are a 'must' in practice are:

a. Consent form (procedural)
b. Professional indemnity insurance and
c. History of allergy (drug, food or other).

Record keeping and documentation has its own advantages apart from legal necessity.

Find out what exactly is patient's or accompanying person/relative's concern and **expectations on the first day of patient's visit** and try to resolve promptly.

Pioneering and successful retaiers such as Harry Gordon Selfridge, John Wanamaker and Marshall Field popularised the motto about:

" THE CUSTOMER IS ALWAYS RIGHT !"

Doctors must appreciate that it applies to clinical practice equally well. This is truer when the analysis of the diagnostian within you must give way to major of the patient—however, stupid it may sound. So we are here essentially to deliver the goods as per requirement assessed by us and expectations held out by the patient.

> **Editorial Comments**
> - This is 'Der Emes' or 'THE TRUTH' whether you were practicing in Biblical era or are practicing in 21st century.

Chapter 10

Hypnosis in Dermatology

JN Dave

"Hypnosis is for Healthier Body and Peaceful Mind"

- **The skin is the mirror of mind.**
- To understand from where nonviral or bacterial skin conditions come from, it is necessary to know the development of skin in embryonic stage. The epidermis and the nervous system originates from ectoderm. So, any imbalance within the nervous system is reflected in the epidermis. This is the reason for hypnosis being so productive in dermatology
- It is the tool with many dermatological applications. It involves guiding the patient into a trance state for specific purpose such as relaxation, pain or pruritus reduction or habit modification.

Hypnosis is the intentional induction, deepening, maintenance and termination of the natural trance state for a specific purpose.

- For medical hypnotherapy, the intent is to reduce suffering, to promote healing or to help the person alter a destructive behavior pattern
- It can be used to increase healthful behaviours, decrease situational stress, needle phobias, controls harmful habits like scratching, provide immediate and long-term analgesia and decrease pruritus
- It can be specially helpful for dealing with skin problems having psychosomatic aspects
- It is not a therapy in and of itself. It's a tool that can be used to cut through psychological behavior, roadblocks to healing
- It is effective for the treatment of dermatological conditions in three specific ways. Firstly, treatment of the root cause, secondly, remission of the symptom and finally through treating the conditioned response to the symptom
- Working with dermatological conditions is one of the most rewarding types of treatment in hypnosis.

Stress
- Stress increases the vulnerability of the autonomic nervous system having a direct effect on the epidermis playing an important role in onset, exacerbation and prolongation of various dermatological conditions
- Autonomic functions can be manipulated using hypnosis and by reducing the stress component of the problem , the symptom itself will reduce.

The list for common dermatological conditions where hypnosis is reasonably useful to decrease symptoms and improving aspects of the condition.

Psoriasis
- Stress plays an important role in the onset, exacerbation and prolongation of psoriasis. Hypnosis has positive effects on psoriasis (Tausk and Whitmore 1999).

Atopic Dermatitis
- Atopic dermatitis resistant to conventional treatment is responsive to hypnosis as an adjuvant therapy. There was reduction in itch, scratching, sleep disturbance and tension. For milder cases of atopic dermatitis, hypnosis was sufficient along with moisturization (Stewart and Thomas 1995).

Acne Excoriee
- Acne excoriee was controlled by using posthypnotic suggestion
- Under hypnosis, the patient was instructed to remember the word "scar" whenever patient wanted to pick his/her face and to refrain from picking by saying "scar" instead. It was the excoriations that resolved, not the underlying acne (Hollander 1959).

Alopecia Areata
- There is a strong correlation between high-stressed reactivity and depression was found in patients with alopecia areata
- Hypnosis can be used to teach patients how to control high-stress reactivity
- It may be more appropriate as a complementary therapy rather than as a primary alternative treatment method for alopecia areata.

Postherpetic Neuralgia
- Improvement in discomfort from herpes simplex eruptions is similar to that of postherpetic neuralgia
- Reduction in the frequency of recurrences of herpes simplex following hypnosis (Bertolino 1983)

- The pain of acute herpes zoster and of post herpetic neuralgia is reduced by hypnosis (Scott 1960).

Lichen Planus
- Both the pruritus and the lesions may be reduced in selected cases using hypnosis as a complementary therapy for lichen planus (Scott 1960).

Rosacea
- In resistant cases of rosacea, especially the vascular blush component where hypnosis was added as a complementary therapy.

Neurodermatitis
Neurodermatitis stayed resolved with up to 4 years of follow-up (Lehman 1978).

Hypnotic Relaxation during Procedures
- A variety of dermatological procedures can produce pain or anxiety in patients. Skin procedures which are painful but usually do not require local anesthetic are moderate-depth chemical peels. Cryodestruction of skin lesions, curettage of molluscum, excision of skin tags, extrusion of comedones, incision and expression of milia, laser treatment of vascular lesions, strong microdesiccation and curettage, incision and drainage of abscesses, laser ablation of skin lesions, liposuction, punch biopsy, shave biopsy, surgical excision and surgical repair. Dermatological procedures that may require conscious sedation include deep chemical peel, dermabrasion, laser resurfacing and extensive liposuction
- All of the above procedures can be augmented by hypnotic relaxation and/or hypnotic analgesia.

STDs
- In cases of genital herpes simplex treated with hypnosis, there was a significant reduction in the number of symptom episodes accompanied by an increase in the number of CD4 and CD8 lymphocytes (Fox et al., 1999)
- HIV phobia
- HIV with decreased CD4 cell count
- Erectile dysfunction and premature ejaculation.

OTHER SKIN CONDITIONS WHERE HYPNOSIS IS HELPFUL
- Verruca vulgaris
- Urticaria
- Congenital ichthyosiform erythroderma

- Dyshidrotic dermatitis
- Erythromelalgia
- Furuncles
- Glossodynia
- Herpes simplex
- Hyperhidrosis
- Ichthyosis vulgaris
- Nummular dermatitis
- Pruritus
- Rosacea
- Trichotillomania
- Vitiligo.

Case 1: Chronic Urticaria

A male patient aged 32 years with chronic urticaria since 2 months was treated with Tab allegra and systemic steroids.

On detailed history and interrogation, he had severe dyspepsia, was suffering from cardioneurosis and was heavy smoker. He was counselled and convinced for hypnosis.

Within 4 sessions, he started reducing the number of cigarettes, his burning pain in abdomen was diminished and supportive antihistaminics were given with Tab. Ranitidine. On completion of 8 sessions on 20 days span he was totally better. Smoking reduced to 4 per day and was maintained on antihistaminic and Tab. Ranitidine.

Eight hypnotic sessions were given in 20 days and 3–4 sessions were given every fortnight, within this period his urticaria totally diappeared.

Tab ranitidine was taken as and when required and he was off the antihistaminic therapy.

Case 2: HIV Phobia

A male patient aged 28 years, staying at Surat, diamond worker had history of CSW exposure for couple of time and developed HIV phobia. As suggested by one of his friend he came to clinic and narrated that from here only I am going to Kankariya lake for suicide.

I talked to him and looking to the severity of his emotional status I took him to deep trance and made few suggestions about life and when he came out of trance after 35 minutes, I again asked about going to Kankariya lake for suicide, he said "sir life is so beautiful, so pleaserous, so joyous and I have responsibility of my wife, child and old parents. I am going home and will see you tomorrow." He was again given 8–10 sessions fortnightly.

N/b: When he came to clinic he had reports of more than 10 laboratories suggestive of HIV -ve and 1–2 reports of weekly +ve HIV.

Chapter 11

Oil Melanosis

JN Dave

CASE NO. 1

- **Age:** 42 years
- **Sex:** Female

Duration of the Disease

11 Months

History

Complain of hyperpigmented lesions over the face.
- H/o application of homemade green-coloured hair oil
- H/o treatment from different private practitioners.

Clinical Examination

Well-defined hyperpigmented patches present over the forehead and sidelocks.

Differential Diagnosis

a. Melasma
b. Riehl's melanosis
c. Postinflammatory hyperpigmentation
d. Photodamage.

Investigations

1. CBC : HB–8.6
2. Wood's lamp: accentuation present

Final Diagnosis

Diffuse facial hypermelanosis (oil).

Management

- Advice to wash face 3–4 times daily with cold water
- Dietary advice to correct anemia (jaggery, walnut, apple, pomegranate, dates, lemon juice)

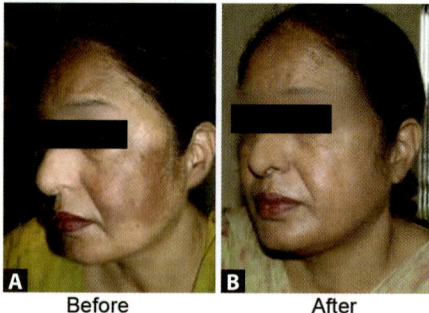

Figs 1A and B: (A) Well-defined hyperpigmented patches present over cheeks and forehead; (B) Excellent response to therapy

- Patient was prescribed Vitamin C supplements and hydroquinone (4%), tretinion (0.025%), fluocionolone acetonide (0.01%) (Figs 1A and B).

> ### Tips
> - Strict advice to avoid using of hair oil
> - Avoid faulty measures like eye rubbing, cosmetic usage, excessive strain nail polishing.
> - Avoid stress
> - Take adequate sleep (7–8 hrs/day).

> ### Editorial Comments
> - Finding aggravating or triggering factors for certain skin diseases is important for its treatment.
> - Simple procedures or habit changing helps in cure of certain skin lesions.

Nail Pitting

CASE NO. 2

- **Age:** 36 years
- **Sex:** Male

Duration of the Disease

2 Years

History

Complain of pitting over right middle finger nail.
- H/o playing carrom
- No h/o involvement of any other finger nails.

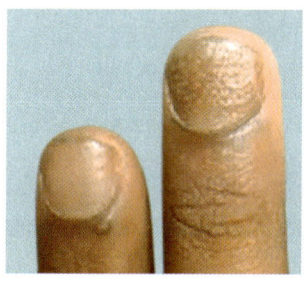

Fig. 2: Multiple, fine pits distributed evenly over the nail plate of right middle finger

Clinical Examination

Well-defined, small fine pittings distributed evenly over the nail plate of right middle finger (Fig. 2).

Differential Diagnosis

a. Psoriasis
b. Alopecia areata
c. Lichen planus.

Investigations

Dermatoscopy.

Final Diagnosis

Traumatic nail injury.

Management

- Avoid trauma
- Use of bandage or artificial acrylic nails while playing carrom
- Moisturize nails using nail moisturizing
- Vitamin D cream massage for five minutes twice daily.

> **Tips**
> - Nail bandaging while playing carrom.

Hair Loss

CASE NO. 3

- **Age:** 26 years
- **Sex:** Female

Marital Status

Unmarried

Duration of the Disease

4 months

History

Complain of diffuse hair loss over the scalp.

- H/o weight reduction programme prior to complaint before 6 months
- H/o stress
- H/o using dove shampoo on alternate day and h/o using conditioner(dove) present.
- No h/o hair loss in family
- No h/o menstrual abnormalities
- No h/o any systemic illness
- No h/o dandruff
- No h/o dye, mehandi, gel application.

Clinical Examination

Diffuse hair loss with thin, lusterless, brisk and black hairs present over the scalp.
- Average calorie intake of patient—1260 calorie/day
- Height—5.4 feets
- Weight—59.6 kgs.

Investigations

1. CBC: HB—10.2%.
2. Dermascopy
   - Sparse hairs present
   - No features suggestive of any hair shaft anomaly (nodes, curls, narrowings, bands, splits, grooves, fracture)
3. Hair pull test: Hair not easily pluckable.

Clinical Appearance

Telogen effluvium (Fig. 3).

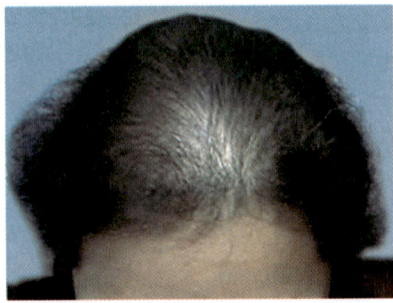

Fig. 3: Diffuse thinning of scalp hair with dry, lusterless hair

Management
- Advice hair wash using cold water
- Dietary advice to correct anemia (jaggery, walnut, apple, pomegranate, dates, lemon juice)
- Proper diet to be taken.

> ***Tips***
> - Avoid faulty measures like ironing, gel or mehandi.
> - Avoid use of conditioner.

Chapter 12

Endurance and Patience

Krina Bharat Patel

What dermatology can teach to all medical students and what wonder dermatology has done on me is an essence of my chapter. The early lessons I learnt from my teachers and which at each and every step my seniors whom I worked with emphasized on; is the art and science of observation and reasoning.

Here I would emphasize on the fact that every patient has something specific and for specific reason—no disease is 'nonspecific' or 'idiopathic'; it's our own zest to delve deep which ultimately may lead us to center of the problem.

This learning has always helped me in arriving at correct diagnosis for difficult to diagnose patients who may have clinical findings which are sometimes described as 'non-specific' or nonexistent and has given me immense satisfaction of touching someone's life for betterment and save my patients from agony of living with skin disease.

Case 1

A 60-year-old male patient came to our OPD for persistent skin lesions of 2 years duration with intractable itching all over body. He was accompanied by a relative with a quiet a big pile of old case papers from various hospitals.

Patient gave history of itchy papules appearing on and off without any seasonal variation. He had no other medical problem and was not taking any medicines except for his skin lesions. He had never taken any alternative medicines in past. His past clinical diagnosis was s/o prurigo nodularis. He was on oral steroids in the dose of 20mg on and off, oral doxycyline 100mg twice per day and topical steroids when he came to us for consultation.

O/E patient had multiple, excoriated papulonodular lesions with postinflammatory hyperpigmentation and hypopigmentation all over body including his face. Scalp, mucosa and palms—soles were unaffected (Figs 1 to 3).

Routine investigations including blood count, liver and renal function tests, X-ray chest, etc. were normal. Skin biopsy

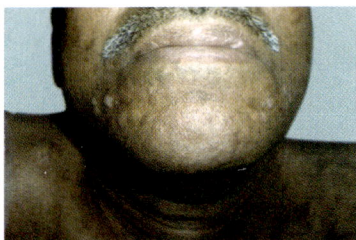

Fig. 1: Papules and excoriated lesions on face

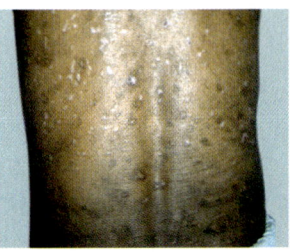

Fig. 2: Post-inflammatory hyperpigmentation and hypopigmentation with few resolving lesions on trunk

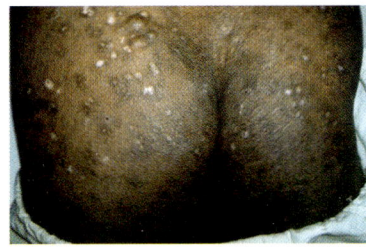

Fig. 3: Excoriated papules, pigmentory changes and few tense blisters on lower back and buttocks

was done from papular lesion on back. Histopathology did not favor diagnosis of prurigo nodularis and was reported as 'nonspecific' findings and need for repeat biopsy. On reviewing the section we found subepidermal split in one of the section which raised some doubts. Patient was advised to stop all oral and topical medicines except oral antihistaminics for some time.

Within 10 days patient came with few new papular lesions and on buttocks he had few tense blisters. Repeat biopsy from the blister showed subepidermal split with minimal inflammatory infiltrate of mixed type. At this stage direct immunofluroscence from perilesional site showed linear deposition of IgG at dermoepidermal junction leading to the final diagnosis of **'prurigo nodularis type of bullous pemphigoid'.**

Bullous pemphigoid is relatively easy to diagnose skin condition for dermatologists but when it presents in its unusual form it poses difficulty. When condition is chronic, clinical picture becomes confusing even more due to various treatments given. At this time stopping all the treatment for a time being and closely observing the patient for development of fresh lesions pays off like in this patient.

Regular oral steroids in tapering doses and topical steroids gave patient relief from his symptoms.

Case 2

A 19-year-old female patient came to skin OPD for recurrent, painful, papulonodular lesions on palms and soles appearing in crops on and off since last 10 years. Skin lesions were associated with high-grade fever and joint pains particularly in ankle, elbow and wrist joints. Her skin lesions were diagnosed as recurrent vasculitis due to unknown etiology and patient was prescribed a course of oral steroids and oral antibiotics whenever she presented with skin lesions.

On examination, patient had multiple erythematous, tender, papules and nodules on dorsa of her hands and feet, as well as sides of palms and soles. There was presence of few traumatic scars on dorsa of her hands (Figs 4 and 5). On thorough examination of entire body single erythematous, asymptomatic plaque with mild scaling was found on extensor of right elbow and generalized xerotic skin was observed (Fig. 6). Patient had history of occasional blood-stained discharge from nose. Patient was generally

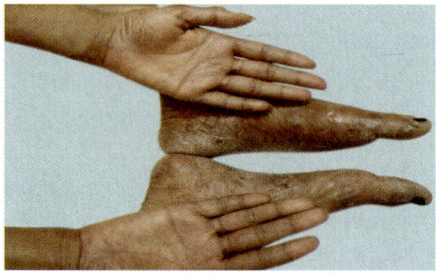

Fig. 4: Papulo-nodular lesions on palms and soles with few crusted and ulcerated lesions

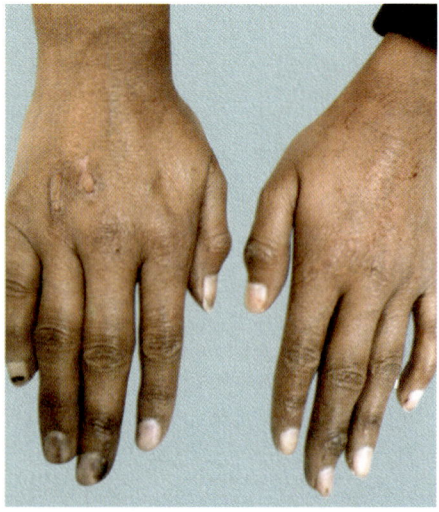

Fig. 5: Shows traumatic lesion and scars on dorsa of hands

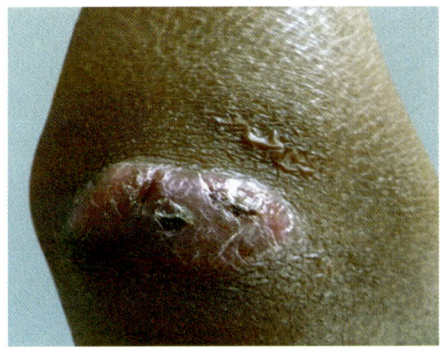

Fig. 6: Single erythematous plaque on elbow with xerosis of skin

malnourished with low body weight for her age and height; which her mother attributed to her chronic illness and reluctance to eat.

Her past history was positive for valvular heart disease for which monthly injection penicillin were given for 12 months. Her medical records suggested mild mitral regurgitation due to rheumatic heart disease. There was no other history of any illness like tuberculosis, hepatitis, etc. No other significant clinical findings were found on general examination. Hematological investigations in past showed persistently low hemoglobin (<9g%) and neutrophilic leucocytosis with each episode of painful lesions associated with fever. Test for RA factor was repeatedly negative, S. ANA was negative twice but pANCA was positive (with no mention of titre) once in past.

As the clinical presentation was curious enough with possibility of systemic vasculitis (Wegner's syndrome or polyarteritis nodosa), routine investigations were advised and skin biopsy was taken from lesion on left leg. While waiting for biopsy report, during follow up-patient presented with fluid-filled lesions on dorsa of her feet which she reported to be due to hot water fomentation which she did due to severe pain (Fig. 7). Suspicious enough for vasculitis right?

On reviewing her H & E section pathologist became skeptical as there was no sign of vasculitis and dermal inflammation showed lots of foamy histiocytes. AFB staining for lepra bacilli showed huge number of bacilli, and was so much exciting for even a pathologist that laboratory called us in closing hours to inform this baffling report and even suggested rebiopsy in case samples have been mixed up! Slit skin smear confirmed the diagnosis with presence of 6+ bacilli.

Now with biopsy reports in hand entire jigsaw puzzle automatically fell at its place.

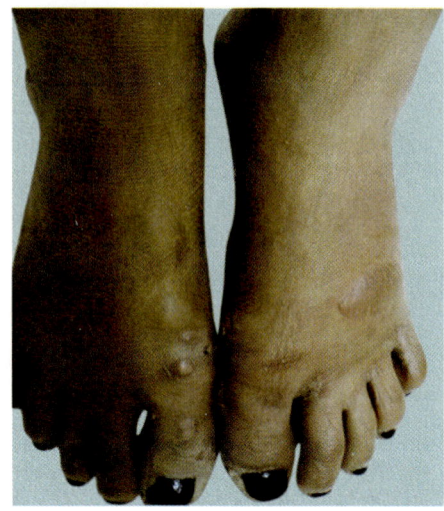

Fig. 7: Blisters developed after hot water fomentation done for relieving pain

12 months of ALT lead to complete resolution of her symptoms and follow-up biopsy showed granular bacilli only; suggesting complete response to therapy. Patient is still under follow-up regularly after 10 months of completion of ALT, with no signs/symptom of recurrence.

This case is a classic example of usefulness of histopathology for skin disorders. Our simple belief of not accepting the diagnosis of vasculitis when everything was not explainable led us to stretch us further and the result was so gratifying. Patient was freed of all her agony of past 10 years within a year of treatment.

> **Editorial Comments**
> - Do not accept when your mind is not convinced. Do not get biased by stamped diagnosis. Always take your call.

Chapter 13

Verruca Plana Treated with Oral Acitretin

Kiran Godse

CASE NO. 1

- **Age (at the presentation of the disease):** 21 years
- **Sex:** Male

Duration of the Disease

2 years

History

- H/O asymptomatic raised lesions over face since 2 years
- H/O gradual increase in number of lesions
- H/O past treatments taken in form of topical creams and TCA application. Patient never had complete clearance of lesions.

Clinical Examination

General examination: Unremarkable.

Cutaneous examination: Multiple, skin coloured to mildly hyperpigmented, thin papules, with flat surface seen over right side of face, including forehead, temple, beard area and neck. Koebnerization positive.

Diagnosis

Verruca Plana.

Investigations

Liver function tests, lipid profile.

Management

Patient was started on oral acitretin 25 mg/day. This was continued for a period of 12 weeks. By 8th–10th week, patient started showing clearance of lesions.

Tips for Managing this Disease

- Acitretin is a good option in recalcitrant warts
- Avoids side effects of local therapy such as pigmentation and scarring after chemical, physical or electric dessication methods
- Useful in cases with widespread or scattered lesions
- Careful patient selection is a must
- Simultaneous use of topical emollients to counteract skin dryness
- Monitoring of lipid profile and LFTs.

> **Editorial Comments**
>
> Newer molecules and their rational use has revolutionazied the way we treat our patients.

Suggested Reading

1. Kaliyadan F, Dharmaratnam AD. Rapid response to acitretin, combined with cryotherapy, for extensive and recalcitrant verruca vulgaris on the scalp. Indian J Dermatol Venereol Leprol. 2011;77:338-40.
2. Krupa Shankar DS, Shilpakar R. Acitretin in the management of recalcitrant warts. Indian J Dermatol Venereol Leprol. 2008;74:393-5.

Molluscum Contagiosum

CASE NO. 2

- **Age (at the presentation of the disease):** 39 years
- **Sex:** Male

Duration of the Disease

6 months

History

Asymptomatic lesions over neck since few months.

Clinical Examination

Multiple, discrete, skin colored to hypopigmented, smooth surfaced, dome-shaped papules, ranging in size from 0.3 mm to 1 cm, few showing central umbilication, seen over anterior neck and lower chin and beard area (Fig. 1).

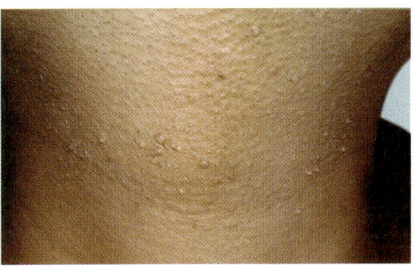

Fig. 1: Patient at presentation, showing multiple skin coloured dome shaped papules over anterior neck.

Diagnosis

Molluscum contagiosum.

Management

Retinoic acid (tretinoin) is a form of chemical ablation which can be self-administered and has been used for treatment of molluscum contagiosum. The method we used was application of topical tretinoin formulation (0.05%), followed by introduction of a 26 gauge needle into the lesion (Figs 2 and 3). This may cause little bleeding, which is controlled with pressure. The lesion turns erythematous and edematous over next few days and soon disappears (Fig. 4). Needling can be performed twice a week and daily application of tretinoin is to be continued. At home, sterile needle may be replaced with clean toothpick for pricking, which usually gives same results and is safer for patients and relatives to use.

With inflammation, molluscum lesions usually disappear within 7–10 days.

For larger lesions tretinoin 0.1% and 21 no. needle can be used.

Side Effects

Rarely, side effects such as erythema, skin drying, peeling and soreness may be observed. However, the incidence of these has been very insignificant in our experience.

Tips for Managing this Disease

- Although molluscum contagiosum is usually an asymptomatic disease, it is contagious and hence should be treated at the earliest
- Left untreated, the lesions typically persist for prolonged periods
- High prevalence in pediatric age group, a factor which influences management

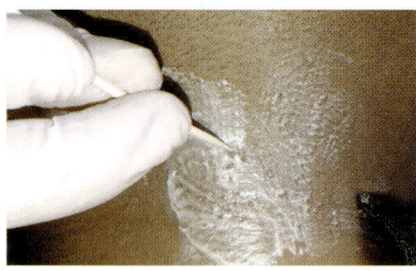

Fig. 2: Patient was treated with topical tretinoin 0.05% cream application, followed by pricking of the molluscum lesions with a toothpick/sterile 26 gauge needle

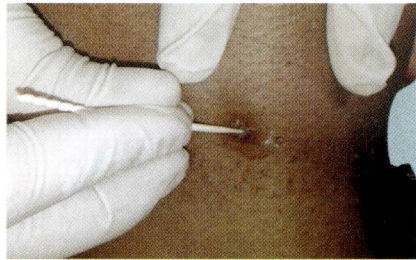

Fig. 3: Needling/pricking of the papule may be followed by minimal bleeding which is controlled with pressure. Erythema may develop followed by resolution of lesions

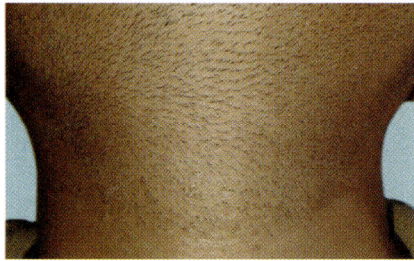

Fig. 4: Patient followed up on day 15 of starting treatment, showing resolution of most of the lesions. No side effects were reported

- Also often seen in immunocompromised/HIV patients, where it presents as giant molluscum
- Commonly administered treatment methods include physical destruction (curettage, electrodessication), chemical destruction (10% KOH application, TCA application) cryotherapy and imiquimod
- However, most of these methods are invasive, or require repeated sittings/administration by the doctor

- Topical tretinoin application followed by needling is a novel method, which can be taught to the patient and self-administered
- It is extremely useful in children, as the method can be taught to parents and done easily at home, absolving the need for office-based painful procedures
- Safe technique, can be used successfully in seropositive patients as it is noninvasive
- Weeks or months of treatment sessions can be converted to days, showing great results with this method.

Advantages

- Noninvasive
- Homebased
- Avoids repeated treatment sessions
- Faster response
- Very-high clearance rate
- No risk of scarring
- Relatively painless
- Easy to perform even in pediatric population
- Easy to use in seropositive patients
- No serious side effects.

> **Editorial Comments**
>
> Simpler and noninvasive methods can be helpful in treatment of some skin disease specially in pediatric age group patients.

Suggested Reading

1. Godse K. Needling in molluscum contagiosum JEurAcadDermatolVenereol. 2006;20(9):1138-9.

Chapter 14

Case Reports on Methotrexate Toxicity

Kirti S Parmar

Dermatologists are quite familiar in using methotrexate for various chronic inflammatory dermatoses; with advancing age changes in serological markers occur leading to methotrexate toxicity-cumulative insult **(case 1)**.

Sometimes patients misinterpret advice about dosage regimen resulting in toxicity **(case 2)**.

Case 1

1. 80-year-old male patient taking regular treatment for psoriasis vulgaris for last 18 years was having following complaints.
2. Fever since 4 days, low grade, on and off, without chills and rigor, relieved by medication.
3. Pedal edema up to knee.
4. H/O scalp scaling present.
5. H/o winter aggravation present.
6. No h/o orogenital lesions, photosensitivity, drug reaction and joint pain.

ON EXAMINATION

- Multiple erythematous plaques over trunk and in the oral lesions (Figs 1 and 2)
- No Lymphadenopathy.

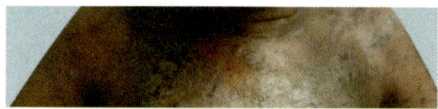

Fig. 1: Multiple erythematous and hyperpigmented plaques with erosions on trunk

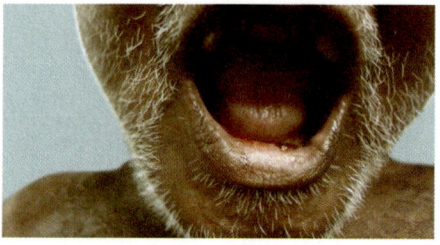

Fig. 2: Erosions in oral cavity

INVESTIGATIONS

	Hb (G/dl)	Total Count (cu/mm)	Platelet Count (cu/mm)
DAY 1	7.13	1889	35000
DAY 2	6.3	920	16000
DAY 3	5.0	800	12000

RENAL FUNCTION TEST

	S.Urea (mg/dl)	S.Creatinine (mg/dl)	S.Sodium (meq/dl)	S.Potassium (meq/dl)
DAY 1	79	1.4	129.7	2.74
DAY 2	40.4	1.16	142.8	2.69
DAY 3	50.1	1.45	140.0	3.00

	S.SGPT (U/L)	S.SGOT (U/L)	S.Bilirubin (mg/dl)	S.Total Protein/Albumin	S.Alp (U/L)	RBS (mg/dl)
DAY 1	28.5	50	4.35	5.12/3.67	87	87
DAY 2	57	90	5.00	4.52/4	100	90
DAY 3	100	200	5.5	5.1/3	304	100

1. Urine culture sensitivity—E.coli isolated
   - Sensitive to imipenam, amikacin, polymixin-B, nitrofurantoin.
2. Blood culture—No organism isolated
3. P.S. for atypical cells—Negative

Differential Diagnosis

1. Sezary syndrome
2. Methotrexate toxicity

From the clinical history and investigation we confirmed our diagnosis and managed the patient with hematologist's advice.

Ongoing Treatment

1. Inj. NS
2. Inj. Dexona 2 cc
3. Inj. Piptaz 4.5 g iv 6 hrly
4. Inj. Vancomycin 1 g iv BD
5. Inj. Avil
6. Inj. Rantac
7. Tab. Metoprolol 25 mg BD
8. Tab. Fe/FA
9. Tab. MV/BC

10. Fusidic acid cream L/A
11. Betamethasone cream L/A
12. Clobetasol+salicylic acid lotion L/A

DIAGNOSIS

1. From above investigation especially pancytopenia we have kept the diagnosis MTX TOXICITY.
2. Patient was referred to Gujarat Cancer Research Institute for further management.

Specific Treatment

1. He was given injection LEUOCOVORIN 15 mg/2 ml diluted in 2 cc water 6 hourly iv for 8 days.
2. Injection FILGRASTIM 300mcg given sc od for seven days.

During specific treatment patient condition gradually improved.

	Hb (Gm/dl)	Total Count (cu/mm)	Pletelet Count (cu/mm)
DAY 6	7.25	3100	88,000
DAY 9	8.00	3500	1,00,000
DAY 12	8.2	7000	1,15,000
DAY 14	8.3	9270	1,87,000

Case 2

1. A 47-years-old female came to our OPD with c/o skin lesions since 6 months.
2. On reviewing history, we found that patient was taking treatment for psoriasis from Rajasthan for last 6 months
3. Patient was given tablet methotrexate 10 mg/week for psoriasis vulgaris, but by mistake she was taking 1 tab/day for last 10 days

ON EXAMINATION

1. Patient was admitted in medical ward for fever and stomatitis.
2. Patient had generalized erythema with scaling and severe erosions in oral cavity.
3. On systemic examination no abnormality found.

She was referred to dermatologist for mucocutaneous involvement.

We reviewed the case, there were no psoriatic lesions on the body, nail showed classical pitting.

INVESTIGATION

1. Hb (G/dl): 8
2. TC (cu/mm): 2600
3. DC (cu/mm): 48/46/2/4
4. Platelets (cu/mm): 18000
5. Blood Sugar (mg/dl): 97
6. S. Urea (mg/dl): 18
7. S. Creat (mg/dl): 0.41
8. S.Na + (meq/dl): 137
9. S.K + (Meq/dl): 4.02
10. Sgot (U/l): 34
11. Sgpt (U/l): 28
12. ALP (U/l): 69
13. S. Protein (g/dl): 5.04
14. S. Albumin (g/dl): 3.10
15. Urine Routine and Micro: NAD
16. ECG: NSR WNL
17. Chest Xray: NAD

Specific Treatment

Patient was on
- Inj. folinic acid IV OD
- Inj. NS 500ml IV BD
- Inj. ceftriaxone (1g) IV TDS
- Inj. metronidazole (500 mg) IV TDS
- Inj. paracetamol (2cc) IV diluted if temp >100
- T. BC/FA 1 OD
- T. dicyclomine 1 SOS

Oral Erosions (Fig. 3)

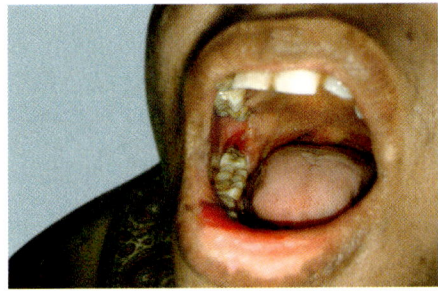

Fig. 3: Multiple oral erosions

Role of Dermatologist

When patients are on methotrexate

Hematologic toxic effects such as pancytopenia represents greatest potential for loss of life due to methotrexate (greatest amount of data in literature is due to rheumatology).

1. Search of identifiable and avoidable risk factors is poor renal function and drug interactions.
2. Vigilant about potential infections, malignancy induction.
3. Consider supplementing folic acid 1–5 mg daily.
4. There are certain group of diseases like chronic inflammatory dermatoses, autoimmune blistering diseases, collagen vascular diseases in which patient has to take regular treatment.

At times complicated life-threatening state requires urgent intervention with intensive care management with multidisciplinary task work.

> **Editorial Comments**
>
> Methotrexate is a magic drug but on the other hand it's a dangerous drug if its intake results in toxicity due to dosage alteration, biochemical parameters alteration.

Chapter 15

Neglected Nevi: A Stitch in Time Saves Nine

Kirti S Parmar

CASE NO. 1

- **Age:** 20 years
- **Sex:** Female

Duration

Since 15 years

History

C/o slightly raised asymptomatic black skin lesions over left side of the forehead for 15 years with irregular folds over scalp and loss of hair on the same side since past 5 years. No history of headache, vomiting, dizziness, loss of consciousness, convulsions, disturbance in speech or vision.

Clinical Findings

Well-circumscribed, pigmented plaque, with a somewhat velvety surface over left side along the hair margin with multiple folds and furrows resembling the surface of the brain with bald patch over the involved area of scalp (Fig. 1).

Digits, toes and nails were found to be normal. No other significant cutaneous or systemic changes were noticed.

Investigations

Complete blood Count, blood sugar levels and endocrine tests were within normal limits. MRI brain and CT scan showed thickening of skin and subcutaneous tissue with multiple folds, underlying bony tissue and structures were normal.

Final Diagnosis

Sebaceous nevus with cutis verticis gyrata.

Treatment History

Nd: YAG laser treatment for sebaceous nevus

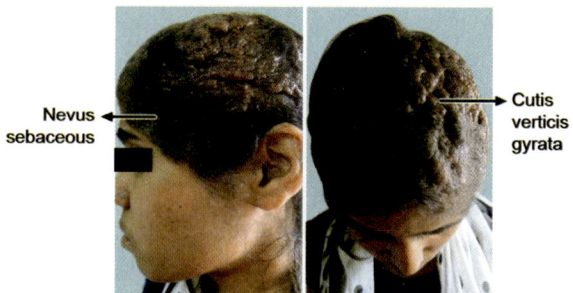

Fig. 1: Lesion on scalp in cutis verticis gyrata type

CASE NO. 2

- **Age:** 15 years
- **Sex:** Male

Duration
Since 15 years

History
C/o slightly pigmented warty streaks and plaques present since birth increasing along the Blashko's line. Patient complained that the lesions have darkened and the surface has become more warty especially over the elbow region since past one year. Associated complaint of nail changes since birth was present with recent worsening.

Clinical Findings
Linear verrucous lesions over forearm and dorsum of hand with plaque like verrucous lesion over elbow was noted over extensor surface of the right hand and back. Tenting of nails in the center with multiple transverse furrows was noted in the middle, ring and little finger (corresponding the site of involvement) (Fig. 2).

Investigation
Complete blood count was normal.

Final Diagnosis
Linear verrucous epidermal nevus.

Treatment History
- RF cautery (after negative HIV test) for the verrucous lesion over the elbow

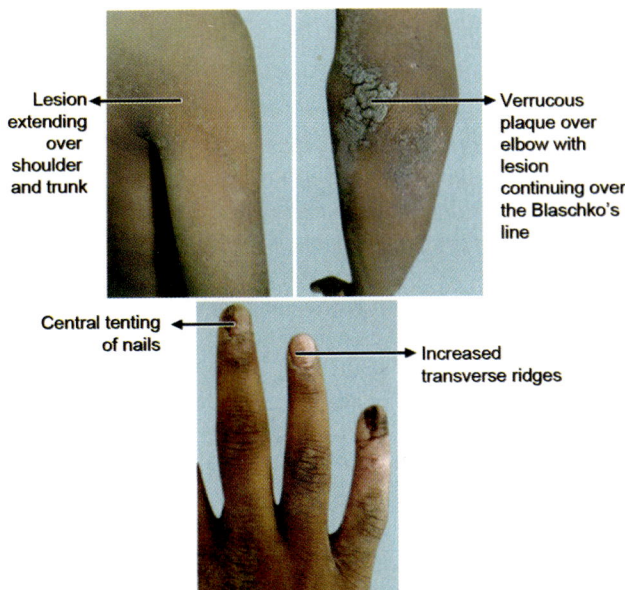

Fig. 2: Lesion in Blaschko-linear distribution

- Cryotherapy along the course of the nevus
- Topical retinoids daily and glycolic acid 70% peel every 3 weeks for the nails.

The occurrence of nevus sebaceous along with other nevi is related to genetic mosaicism and the shape and distribution of the nevus is determined by the stage at which mosaicism has arisen. Malignancy probably develops only in longstanding or neglected lesions but exceptionally can be a source of mortality. Rapid, circumscribed enlargement or ulceration should arouse suspicion of malignant transformation.

Usually hemangiomas are known for hyperplasia but in this case nevus sebaceous shows secondary hyperplasia in the form of development of cutis verticis gyrata which is unsightly and hard to manage.

Thus, early treatment should always be considered if patient presents at an earlier age. Lesions within the scalp may be difficult to follow clinically and extirpation will prevent the development of occult secondary changes. For facial lesions, consideration should be given to excision during childhood, before the development of secondary verrucous alteration, at a time when the risk of scarring is reduced compared to adulthood. The excisional margins can be minimal.

> **Tips**
> - Nevus is the Latin word for 'maternal impression' or 'birthmark' and indicates a circumscribed, nonneoplastic skin or mucosal lesion, usually present at or soon after birth and fixed.

Linear verrucous epidermal nevus is usually easily managed. Large lesions may require multistage, multimodality procedures, adapted according to anatomical site. It is suggested that increased hormonal activity may potentiate the growth of these lesions, as growth spurt is often noted at puberty.

Verrucous hyperplasia over elbow occurred mostly due to repetitive friction at the site with time.

Additional segmental manifestations like lipomatosis, fibromas, vascular malformations (frequently with an arteriovenous component) and asymmetric overgrowth of the soft tissues and bones may be present either locally or as a part of syndromes. Nail changes can thus be attributed to increased vasculature and nail bed proliferation leading to tenting of nail plates and formation of transverse ridges.

> **Editorial Comments**
> - Nevus as we know is very common but it has to be very closely monitored for any secondary changes which can be suggestive of malignant change.
> - Better to excise nevus at early stage as a step of prevention.

Chapter 16

AIDS Cholangiopathy

Keyur Shah, Neetisha Agarwal

F/45 years presented to general surgeon in 7/08 with c/o
- Pain in abdomen on and off
- Fullness of abdomen
- Anorexia since 5-6 months
- Weight loss
- Vomiting occassional.

H/o hysterectomy in 1991, h/o 2 blood transfusions received.

General Examination

- Anemia+
- No icterus
- Generalised mild tenderness in abdomen
- No hepatosplenomegaly.

Investigations

- Hb: 10.5 g%
- TC: 3200
- DC: Polymorphs—71, Lymphocytes—28
- ESR: 95
- PC: 1.80 lacs
- S. bilirubin: 0.95 (D=0.45, I=0.5)
- SGPT: 25.2
- S.ALK.PO4: 335
- Urine: NAD
- S.creat: 1.0
- HBsAg: Negative.

USG Abdomen

- Dilatation of IHBR with extrahepatic CBD (11.2 mm) till the lower end, possibility of the stricture at the lower end CBD.
- Gallbladder: Moderately distended. No calculi, no bladder wall thickening
  Referred to gastroenterologist.
  Advised for CT abdomen with contrast.

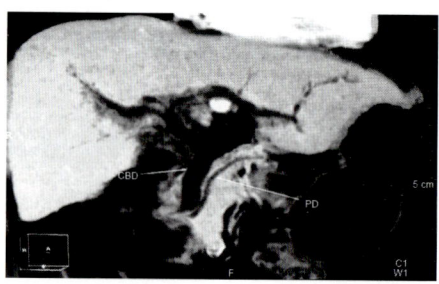

Fig. 1: CT scan changes in liver and gallbladder

CT Abdomen with Contrast
- CBD dilated (10 mm).
- Stricture (concentric wall thickening) of lower end of CBD (Fig. 1). No focal or diffuse hypo or hyperintense SOL seen.

Treatment
- Tab. buscopan
- Tab. ursocol
- Tab. pantocid
- Liq. ulgel

Follow-up after 2 weeks
- Mild relief in c/o
- Abdominal pain: Present
- Anorexia persisted
- Fullness of abdomen present.

MRCP: (25/11/08)
- Dilated IHBR in both lobes of liver.
- Lt. hepatic duct dilated (6 mm)
- Common hepatic duct (11mm), Common bile duct (13mm) dilated.
- CBD shows gradual tapering near ampulla.

Clinical Diagnosis: Cholangiopathy (? Benign)
- Plan: ERCP
- Pre ERCP screening: HIV positive
- Referred to HIV consultant. ERCP postponed.

Patient followed up with:
- Abdominal pain (more in Rt.upper quadrant)
- Fullness of abdomen
- Weight loss
- Anorexia
- Low-grade fever occasionally
- Vomiting occasionally.

General Examination
- Anemia +
- Mild oral candidiasis
- Per Abdomen: Mild tenderness in right hypochondrium

Investigations
- Hb: 9.5
- TC: 3900
- DC: P65L30
- ESR: 65
- S.Creat: 0.62
- S.Bil: 1.1(D=0.6,I=0.5)
- SGPT: 40
- SGOT: 37
- S.ALPO4: 550
- S. lipase: 137
- Western Blot: HIV 1
- CD4: 35 (16%)
- CD8: 281(80%).

Differential Diagnosis
- AIDS cholangiopathy (cryptosporidia, CMV)
- Viral hepatitis
- Mycobacterial infection of liver: TB, MAC
- Drugs: bactrim, INH, RFM, dapsone, ketoconazole
- Lymphoma.

Treatment
- Tab. nizonide: 500 mg bd x 6 weeks
- HAART: TDF (Tenofovir)+ FTC (emtricitabine) + EFV (EFAVIRENZ) (1 tab/day)
- Tab. bactrim 1od.

Follow-up after 15 days
- Asymptomatic
- No abdominal pain
- Appetite improved
- Weight gain of 3 kg. (35–38 kg)
- S. Alpo4: 250.
- Ct. nizonide, viraday, bactrim for 1 month.

Follow-up after 6 weeks
- Asymptomatic
- No abdominal pain
- Weight gain of 2 kg (38–40 kg)
- CD4: 75 (19%)
- S.Alpo4: 150.

Follow up MRCP
- No dilatation of CBD (7mm), IHBR, EHBR.

Measurement of Biliary ducts
- Pre Treatment Post Treatment
- Left Hepatic duct: 6mm Left hepatic duct: 2mm
- CBD: 13mm CBD: 7.4mm
- MPD: 2mm MPD: 2.1mm

Final Diagnosis
- Cryptosporidial Cholangiopathy in AIDS patient.

Review of Literature-AIDS Cholangiopathy
- Indian Academy of Clinical Medicine, Vol:7, No.1, Jan-Mar, 2006
- NEJM 2002;346:1723
- Clin. Microbiol. Rev 1999;12:554
- Clin Infect Dis. 2001;32:331.

Discussion

AIDS Cholangiopathy
- Biliary syndrome in AIDS pt.
- 1st described by Cello in 1989
- Estimated incidence in AIDS pt: 45%.

DIAGNOSIS
- AIDS cholangiopathy.

Cause
- Cryptosporidiosis ⎫
- CMV   ⎬ Most common
- Microsporidia, Cyclospora, Isospora ⎪
- MAC   ⎭
- Salmonella ⎫ Uncommon
- Candida   ⎭

Pathogenesis: Unclear
- Pathogen-induced cholangiocyte apoptosis and periductal inflammation
- Direct infection of biliary epithelium—not reported.

Clinical Features
- Abdominal pain: Rt. upper quadrant
- Diarrhea (acute/chronic) 90–95%
- Fever with chills
- Jaundice—uncommon (<5%).

Investigations
- Markedly raised S.Alpo4: (4–5 fold)
- Normal/mild elevation of SGPT, S.Bilirubin
- CD4 <50
- USG/MRCP: Intrahepatic and CBD dilatation, terminal stenosis with wall thickening
- Stool: oocyst of cryposporidia.

Prognosis
- Without treatment, median survival: 9 months
- Involvement of other system: GI, skin, CNS s/o poor prognosis
- S.Alpo4 is good indicator for prognosis
- Cryptosporidial cholangitis is the only and very-late presentation of HIV infection
- Cryptosporidial cholangitis without diarrhea.

Treatment
- None antimicrobials proven successful
- Paromomycin: 500 qds x 4 weeks
- Nitazoxanide: 500 bd x 6 weeks
- Azithromycin: 1200 od x 4 weeks
- HAART is the only treatment.

Chapter 17

CD4 and Viral Load Discordance

Keyur Shah, Neetisha Agarwal

What We Know
- HIV science: Evolving, 22 years old
- Many mysteries solved: Virus, pathogenesis, laboratory investigations, treatment
- What to start? When to start? When to change?
- Life-threatening infection–chronic infection
- CD4 and viral loads are two surrogate markers to assess the success of HAART
- Viral load: Long-term risk
- CD4: Short-term risk
- Successful HAART
  - Viral load $\rightarrow$ undetectable at max. 48 weeks
  - CD4 $\rightarrow$ gradually$\uparrow$
- If viral load is not undetectable at 48 weeks $\rightarrow$? 1st line failure–ARV resistance assay to plan 2nd line ARV.

What We Don't Know
- Viral load is undetectable but CD4 after initial improvement, started falling gradually
- ARV resistance is not possible as viral load is undetectable.

Success $\rightleftarrows$ Failure

'More you explore, more you get confused'.

Case 1
- M/45 years, Western Blot proven HIV-1 positive in 2001.
- CD4 nadir: 4
- HAART: d4T+3TC+NVP started
- Highest CD4: 268 (2004)
- Irregular HAART, CD4: 138 (2005)
- d4T+3TC+NVP $\rightarrow$ AZT+ddI+IDV/r
- Irregular HAART
  Presented in Aug. 2008 with
- Carbamazepine induced TEN (for dental neuralgic pain).

- CD4: 45 (8%)
- CD8: 328 (62%)   } ART Failure
- CD4/CD8: 0.14
- Viral load: 580947
- AZT+ddI+IDV/r → TDF+FTC+LPV/r

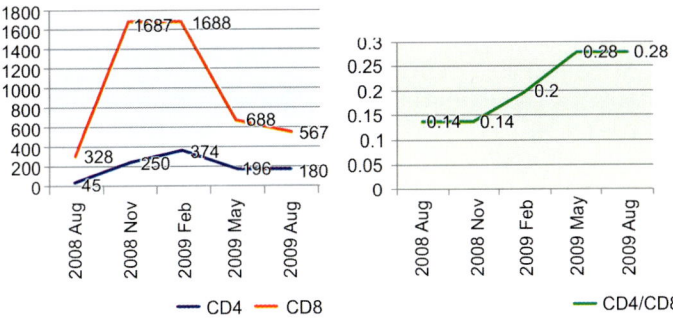

Fig. 1: Charts showing CD4 and CD8 discordance

	8/08	11/08	2/09	5/09	8/09
CD4	45 (8%)	250 (12%)	374 (16%)	196 (14%)	180 (13%)
CD8	328 (62%)	1687 (81%)	1668 (80%)	688 (49%)	567 (46%)
CD4/CD8	0.14	0.14	0.20	0.28	0.28
Viral Load	580947	388 copies			<53 copies

Case 2

- M/33 years, Western Blot proved HIV 1 positive (4/08) screening for fever
  - CD4: 93 (9%)
  - CD8: 834 (81%) d4T+ } 3TC+EFV
  - CD4/CD8: 0.11
- 8/08: restricted elbow movement with swelling Koch's synovitis
  - CD4: 312 (18%)
  - CD8: 1278 (72%) } IRIS-Koch's synovitis
  - CD4/CD8: 0.25

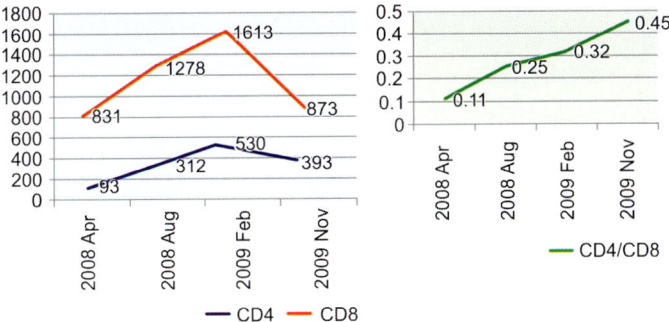

Fig. 2: Charts showing CD4 and CD8 discordance

	4/08	8/08	2/09	11/09
CD4	93 (9%)	312 (18%)	530 (23%)	393 (18%)
CD8	831(81%)	1278(72%)	1613 (70%)	873 (40%)
CD4/CD8	0.11	0.25	0.32	0.45
Viral load				<53 copies

Case 3

- M/58 years, Western Blot proved HIV 1 positive since 1997
- H/o TB pericardial effusion in 2004
- CD4 nadir: 90
- HAART: AZT+3TC+EFV (2004)
- Compliance: Questionable

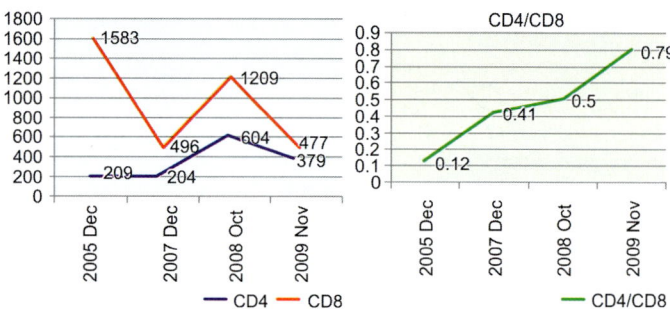

Fig. 3: Charts showing CD4 and CD8 discordance

	12/05	12/07	10/08	11/09
CD4	209 (10.2%)	204 (28%)	604 (30%)	379 (27%)
CD8	1583 (67.4%)	496 (68%)	1209 (60%)	477 (34%)
CD4/CD8	0.12	0.41	0.5	0.79
Viral Load		8481 copies	<53 copies	
HAART		TDF+FTC+LPV/r		

Case 4

- M/48 years, k/c/o NHL 2 1/2 years back, 6 chemotherapy taken

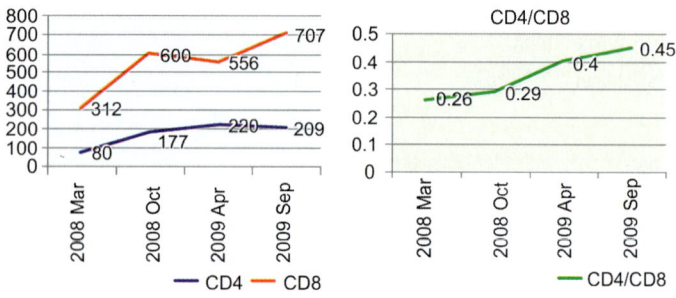

Fig. 4: Charts showing CD4 and CD8 discordance

- Diagnosed HIV 1 + (Western Blot proved) in 2006
- CD4: 98
- HAART: AZT/3TC for 2 1/2 years.

	3/08	10/08	4/09	10/09
CD4	80 (11%)	177 (12%)	220 (14.6%)	209 (11.7%)
CD8	312 (43%)	600 (40%)	556 (37.06%)	707 (26%)
CD4/CD8	0.26	0.29	0.4	0.45
Viral load	65789 copies			<53 copies
HAART	TDF+FTC+EFV			

Case 5

- M/49 years, Western Blot proved HIV 1 + since 2 years. Presented with fever, weight. loss, cough, anorexia
- X-ray chest s/o pulmonary Koch's
- 4 drugs AKT started
- CD4 nadir: 35 (7%)
- HAART started 15 days after AKT. (TDF+FTC+EFV).

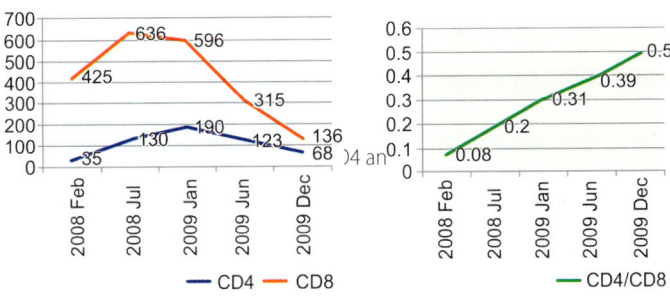

	22/2/08	17/7/08	1/1/09	1/6/09	22/12/09
CD4	35 (7%)	130 (16%)	190 (22%)	123 (16%)	68 (18%)
CD8	425 (86%)	636 (78%)	596 (69%)	315 (41%)	136 (36%)
CD4/CD8	0.08	0.2	0.31	0.39	0.5
Viral load	2598709		<53 copies		<53 copies

Discordant Response

- Failure to achieve all of the therapeutic goals—clinical, immunological, virological—is referred to as a discordant response.

Response to ART	Grabar 2000 N=2236	Moore 2005 N=1527	Tan 2007 N=404
Virological and immunological	48%	56%	71%
Discordant: Only immunological	19%	12%	16%
Discordant: Only virological	17%	15%	9%
No treatment response	16%	17%	5%

Risk Factors for Discordant Response
- Low CD4 at baseline
- Old age (due to thymus degeneration)
- Intravenous drug user
- Concomitant immuno/myelosuppresive drugs
- Certain antiretroviral regimen: TDF+ddI, AZT containing regimen.

Unanswered Questions
What is the reason for this discordance?
- Known phenomenon
- No specific reason

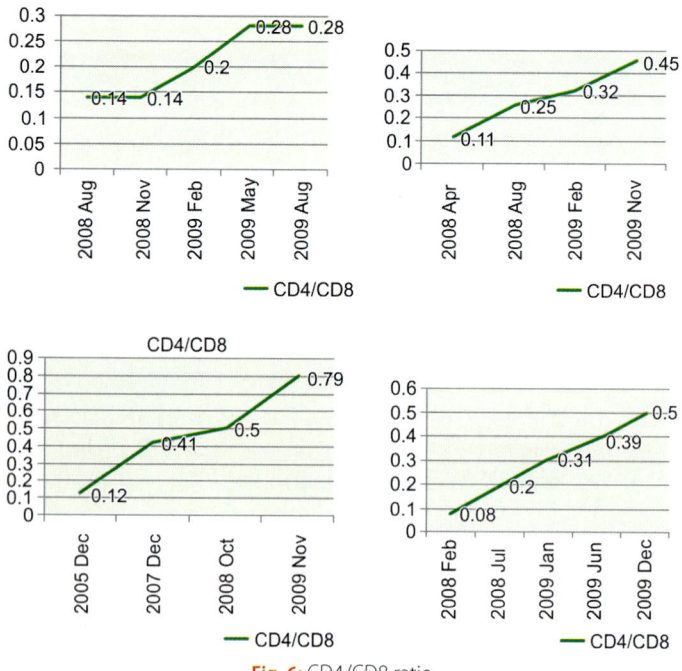

Fig. 6: CD4/CD8 ratio

- Hypothesis: Involvement of LN → distortion of LN architecture → fibrosis of LN → LN exhaustion → no more CD4 production
- Any relation with OI (3pts with tuberculosis, 1 pt with NHL)
- Change in HAART solve the problem?
  - Change of HAART to LPV/r → better CD4 response (few studies) but not proved
- Should we continue OI prophylaxis?
  - Yes
- What to monitor?
  - CD4   --CD4/CD8
  - CD4%   --Viral load

Conclusion

- Absolute CD4 or CD4% can give false idea about success/failure of HAART.
- CD4/CD8 is an answer in such discordant situation.
- Success ↔ Failure.

History of ART

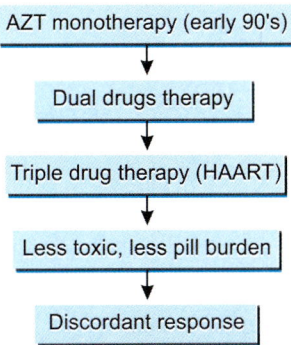

'Enjoy Your Success Till It Proves To Be A Failure'

Editorial Comments

- Though HAART has shown a great success in managing HIV, there are so many unmet needs and unknown challenges that clinicians managing PLHA patients come across.

Chapter 18

VZV Encephalitis with IRIS in PML

Keyur Shah, Neetisha Agarwal

- M/26 years, unmarried graduate presented in Nov. 2006 with complains of
    - Weakness in Rt UL and LL
    - Slurred speech
    - Fever on and off × 1 month after herpes zoster
    - Loss of memory
    - Impaired concentration
- Referred to neurologist
- Investigations ordered:
    - ANA–Negative
    - Vit B12—541.2 (211-911)
    - MRI brain with contrast s/o leukodystrophy
- Treatment given:
    - Prednisolone 1mg/kg with antiepileptic with multivitamins × 15 days
- Not improved, ordered for ELISA for HIV and found reactive
- H/o herpes zoster twice.
    - 1st episode: 2 years back
    - 2nd episode: 3 months back
- H/o weight loss (approximately 5 kg. in 3 months).

Examination
- Vital signs:
    - Temp: raised (102°F)
- Mild oral candidiasis.

Systemic Examination
- Recent amnesia, ataxia, partial aphasia
- Rt. facial weakness, Rt. UL and LL weakness
- Cerebellar sign +
- DTR: Brisk plantar
- Sensation: Normal.

Clinical Diagnosis

- Encephalitis (varicella zoster virus or toxoplasmosis)
    OR
- PML (progrssive multifocal leukoencephalopathy)
Patient was advised for admission for further investigations and treatment.

Investigations

- Hb: 12.7g%
- TC: 5400
- DC: P63L34
- ESR: 45 (1sthr)
- SGPT: 34
- S.creat: 1.02
- Na: 132, K: 3.5
- CPK total: 55, LDH: 62
- CD4: 46/cmm
- CSF:
    - Protein: 26
    - Sugar: 56
    - Total cell: 2 (100%L)
    - AntiHerpes zoster IgG: 24 EU/ml (Normal: 1-10), anti-herpes zoster IgM: 8EU/ml (Normal: 1-10).

MRI Brain with Contrast (27/11/06)

Left temporo-occipital paraventricular fairly large abnormal signal intensity changes in white matter and small area of abnormal mild T2W prolongation in right occipital white matter also. Postcontrast no abnormal enhancement (Fig. 1).

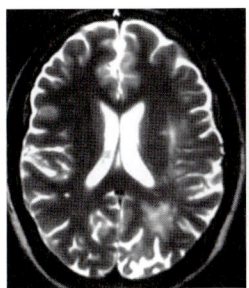 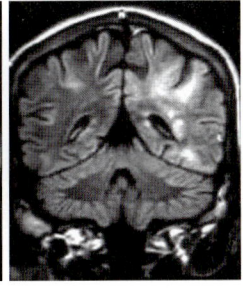

Fig. 1: MRI findings

FINAL DIAGNOSIS

- VZV encephalitis (? PML) in immunocompromised patient (CD4 = 46).

Treatment
- IV acyclovir—10mg/kg 8 hrly × 14 days
- PCP prophylaxis
- HAART: AZT+3TC+LPV/r
- Pt was discharged after 14 days (27/12).

On Discharge
- Pt was not improved clinically.
- Weakness persist in both Rt UL and LL
- Vision is compromised (Rt>Lt)
- Partial aphasia persist.

Reviewed Diagnosis
VZV encephalitis with PML

Follow-up (After 1 Month)
- Gradual deterioration
- Power: Gd:2 to Gd:0
- Vision: Completely blind in both eyes (ophthalmic examination s/o retrobulbar neuritis)
- Complete aphasia.

F/UP MRI (29/1/2007)
Signal intensity markedly increase in left posterior cerebrum paraventricular region and moderately increase on right posterior temporo-paraventricular region. Splenium of corpus callosum, left infrathalamic mid brain and left anterior temporoparietal region are new areas of abnormality.

Finding show radiological deterioration and possibility of PML likely (Fig. 2).

29/1/2007: (After 1 Month of HAART)
- CD4: 263 (15%),
- CD8: 1421 (81%),
- CD4/CD8: 0.18.

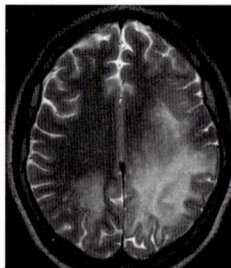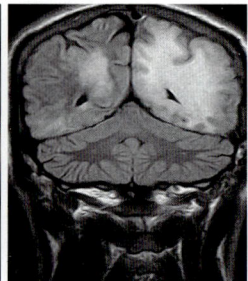

Fig. 2: MRI findings in follow up visit

Treatment
- Systemic steroid (prednisolone 1mg/kg) + HAART (AZT+3TC+LPV/r)
- Gradual improvement noticed after 1 week.

Diagnosis
Immune reconstitution inflammatory syndrome (IRIS) with PML in VZV encephalitis.

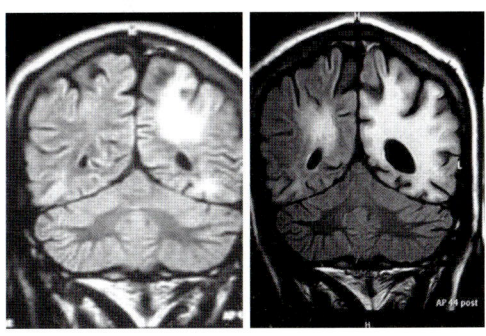

Pretreatment MRI   Post-treatment MRI

Fig. 3: Pre- and post-treatment MRI changes

After 1 1/2 Months
- Power: Gd0 to Gd3
- Vision: Completely blind to 4/6
- Speech: Mute to partial aphasia
- Case is presented for its rarity.
  - VZV encephalitis is rare
  - PML is uncommon
  - Both rare conditions occur in same patient at the same time.

Review of Literature: PML
Clinical course and prognostic factors of progressive multifocal leukoencephalopathy in patients treated with highly active antiretroviral therapy.

    Clinical Infectious Diseases. 2003;36:1047-52.

Chapter 19

Case Reports

Keyur Shah, Neetisha Agarwal

Case History 1

35-year-old married businessman reported for:
- Skin lesion on face suggestive of Hansen's diseases (borderline tuberculoid) and
- Herpes zoster left T12
- Screened for HIV on clinical ground and found HIV-1 reactive.

INVESTIGATIONS

HIV Combo Assessment

Date	Symptoms	CD4 %	Abs. CD4 count	HIV-1 RNA
04.02.2003	Asymptomatic	19.8	299	18,843
18.07.2003	Asymptomatic	19.6	265	14,325
09.01.2004	Asymptomatic	19.0	146	18,465
05.03.2004	Asymptomatic	24.2	281	24,914
11.06.2004	Asymptomatic	19.3	232	45,473

Treatment Plan
- Counselling and under observation
- To postpone HAART.

Reasons for Presentation
1. Herpes zoster has high positive predictive value for HIV infection.
2. Reactivation of Hansen's disease in HIV infection.
3. HAART is lifelong treatment today, it is advisable to postponed. It as long as possible.

Note: Types of HIV Screening
a. Voluntary
b. Anonymous

c. Mandatory (blood/semen/organ donor)
  d. Perinatal
  e. Clinical suspicion
  f. High-risk behavior (IVDU, STD, CSW, multiple transfusion, truck driver).

Case Histroy 2
On 31st January 2004
- 40-year-old married male self-employed based at Belgaum
- C/O Fever, swelling in right side of neck (lymph node enlargement).

Investigations: 31st January 2004
- Complete blood count—Normal
- ESR—4
- Malarial Parasites—Not detected
- Urine examination—Normal
- Sputum examination—AFB not seen
- Renal Profile—Normal
- Liver Profile—Normal except SGOT 101 and SGPT 95
- VDRL—Negative
- HBsAg—Negative
- HIV 1 and 2 –Positive
- USG of abdomen and plevis within normal limits but Multiple enlarge lymph nodes are seen in the neck on right side which showed evidence of internal necrosis.
- Lymph node biopsy—Necrotizing granulomatous lymphadenits—Tubercular, ZN stain—Many acid-fast bacilli seen
- CD 4%—6.16 ↓
- Absolute CD4 count—44 ↓
- HIV 1 RNA—2,65,339 copies/ml.

Treatment Given
- ZDV + 3TC + NVP

Admission by 2nd Consultant (6th February)
- **C/O** PUO, cough, weakness
- **CT scan of chest, abdomen and pelvis:** Enlarged subcarinal lymph nodes, few tiny focal lesions in spleen. Possible diagnosis of TB or lymphoma.

Treatment Given
1. R + H + E + S
2. D4T (stavudine) + 3TC (lamivudine) + NFV (nelfinavir).

Admission by 3rd Consultant (3rd April 2004)
Investigations
- **C/o** PUO, weakness
- **Complete Hemogram**—Normal
- **Malarial parasites**—Not seen
- **Widal Test**—Negative
- **Liver function test**—Normal
- **Antibody to hepatitis C**—Negative
- **CD4 %**—11.8
- **Absolute CD 4 count**—420
- **HIV-1 RNA copies**—33,709.

Treatment Given
- S + R + H + E +Z
- Fluconazole
- Bactrim DS
- No ART.

Follow-up on June 7, 2004
- Asymptomatic.

Investigation
- Complete blood count—Normal
- Liver function test—Normal
- Serum uric acid— 11.2 mg/dl
- CD4 %—7 ↓
- Absolute CD 4 count—145 ↓
- HIV—1 RNA copies—54,840 ↑
- CT scan of chest: Few enlarged mediastinal lymph nodes (no central necrosis)
- CT scan of abdominal and pelvis : Few small nonenhancing splenic lesions seen.
- Bone marrow biopsy : No evidence of lymphoma
- Cervical lymph node biopsy : T cell Lymphoma (CD 20, CD 3 and CD43 marker positive).

Final Impression
T Cell lymphoma.

Treatment Planned
AKT (H + E) + HAART (SQV-Saquinavir + RTV-Ritonavir + ZDV-Zidovudine+3TC)+BactrimDS+Chemotherapyforlymphoma (CHOP—Cyclophosphamide, doxorubicin, vincristine, adriamycin, prednisolone).

Reasons for Presentation

1. PUO as presenting symptom of HIV infection.
2. TB is commonest OI (Opportunistic Infection) responsible for PUO.
3. TB should receive adequate induction phase of AKT.
4. There is no hurry to initiate HAART.
5. There should be strong clinical suspicion for diagnosis of lymphoma, both TB and lymphoma can coexist.
6. Lymphoma is HIV defining illness.
7. HAART should be initiated preceding/simultaneously with chemotherapy for lymphoma.
8. Serum uric acid elevation in symptomatic HIV individuals is not uncommon.

Case History 3

- 30-years-old graduate bachelor self-employed
- Detected HIV seropositive in 1997 during health camp.
- Detected HCV seropositive in 2002 during Hemophilia Society screening
- Severe factor VIII deficiency (<one)
- Recurrent hemarthrosis
- Asymptomatic (HIV infection).

Investigations

- CXR—WNL
- USG—mild splenomegaly
- CD4 %—25.4
- Absolute CD4 count—620
- Hb—12.3
- Platelet—43,400
- SGOT—113
- SGPT—113
- GGT—93
- Total bilirubin—0.9
- Total Protein—9.2
- Albumin – 3.9
- HCV RNA copies 800,000 and genotype 3.

Impression

- Hemophilic having HIV and HCV confection + ITP (idiopathic thrombocytopenia) + chronic hepatitis (liver biopsy difficult) + immunologically stable.

Tips

- HIV science: More you explore, more you get confused
- Pyrexia of unknown origin is the commonest presentation of HIV/AIDS
- Tuberculosis is the commonest opportunistic infection
- Lymphoma is the commonest malignancy in HIV/AIDS but many times mistreated as TB
- Rare is rare but can be present in HIV/AIDS, e.g: AIDS cholangiopathy, VZV encephalitis
- Though CD4 is good marker to know efficacy of anti retroviral drugs, viral load is an answer to prove drug failure
- Do not start HAART in hurry. HAART is an art.

Editorial Comments

- HIV is such a condition which can change the presentation of certain disorders whether systemic or cutaneous
- Treatment of underlying disease along with HIV is important but utmost care should be taken to prevent IRIS or any other drug interaction.

Chapter 20

Trichofolliculoma Presenting as Verrucous Growth

Neela Patel

CASE NO. 1

- **Age:** 75 years
- **Sex:** Male

Duration of the Disease

4 months

History

A 75-year-old male presented with skin lesion on nose for 4 months. H/o trauma on the nose before 6 months. Patient had taken treatment for it but didn't improve.

Clinical Examination

Well-defined, skin-colored firm, dry, nontender, verrucous growth approximatoly 4 × 5 cm in size present over nose involving both ala of nose and extending to left cheek (Fig. 1). Nasal mucosa and oral mucosa were normal.

Submental, submandibular, preauricular lymph nodes were not palpable.

Systemic Examination

RS, CVS, CNS normal.

Provisional Differential Diagnosis

a. TVC
b. SCC.

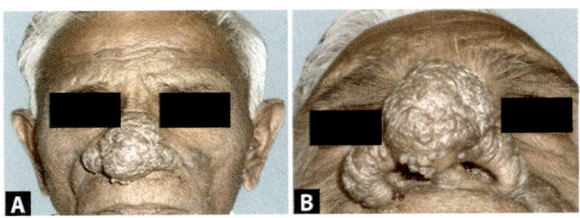

Fig. 1: Verrucous lesion on nose

Investigations

TC ↑ (17000/cmm), differential count: (88/10/1/1), all routine investigations were within normal limit, Mantoux test was negative. Chest X-ray, X-ray local part and USG abdomen were normal.

Patient was referred to plastic surgery department for excision of the lesion and excised lesion was sent for Histopathological examination.

EPIDERMIS shows focal area of hyperplasia. Dermis shows numerous cystic spaces lined by squamous epithelial cells. Cavity contains keratinized horny material and Fragments of hair shaft in some. Marked chronic inflammatory infiltrate surrounding cysts are also seen.

Multiple yet well-differentiated hair follicle radiating from the wall of cysts are present in the dermis.

Epithelial strands interconnect the secondary hair follicles. Epithelial strands differentiate in the direction of outer root sheath so peripheral cell row is arranged in palisaded manner.

Histopathological findings are suggestive of tumor of epidermal appendage with follicular differentiation most probably trichofolliculoma (Figs 2 and 3).

Final Diagnosis

Trichofolliculoma presenting as verrucous growth.

Management

Excision of the lesion was done.

Tips for Managing this Disease

Sometime clinical picture does not resemble the classical skin lesion. We require deep excisional serial biopsy for confirmation of diagnosis.

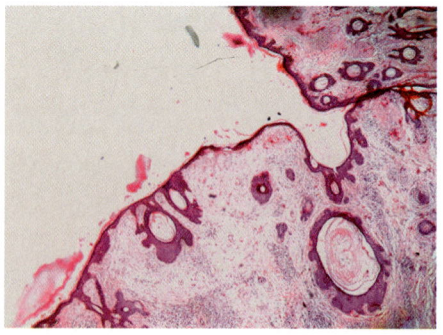

Fig. 2: 4X Showing numerous cystic spaces containing keratinous material in dermis

Trichofolliculoma Presenting as Verrucous Growth

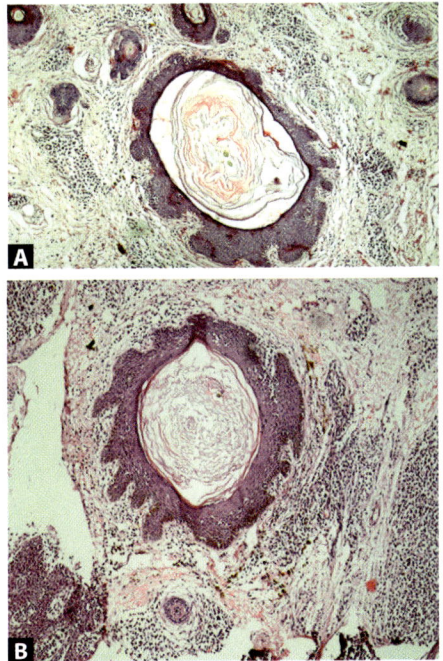

Figs 3A and B: 10X Showing radiating secondary hair follicles from primary cyst wall

Editorial Comments

Common looking skin lesion on atypical site, with atypical presentation and resistant to routine treatment should always be taken as atypical skin disease which has to be proved by HPE or other related tests.

# Chapter 21

Acute Myeloid Leukemia

Neela V Bhuptani

CASE NO. 1

- **Age:** 64 years
- **Sex:** Male

Duration

7 months

History

C/o of multiple skin-colored to reddish elevated itchy lesions over scalp, face, upper back and chest since 7 months. Patient had taken treatment from many private dermatologists in form of systemic and topical antifungal and steroids. Patient had benign prostatic hypertrophy since 4 years and past history of extra-pulmonary TB before 13 years.

Clinical Findings

Multiple skin-colored to erythematous shiny, nontender, firm papules and nodules (follicular and nonfollicular) with gray scaling were present over scalp, face, upper chest and back. Left cervical lymph nodes were palpable.

Various Differentials

Seborrheic dermatitis, pityrosporum folliculitis, demodicidosis, CTCL, cutaneous manifestation of internal malignancy, sarcoidosis and papular tuberculids were considered as per clinical presentation and patient was treated symptomatically but was not much relieved.

Investigations

All investigations were normal on presentation. The subsequent investigations on follow-up (3rd follow-up) were as follows:

- Hb—8.8 g/dl
- TC—25,400 cells/cumm
- DC—30/23/3/7/00
- ESR—46 mm/1st hr.

Peripheral smear: Shift to left with myelocytes along with other myeloid cells (blasts—00, promyelocyte—00, myelocyte—02, metamyelocytes—07, band cells—06).

Histopathology

Thinned-out epidermis with dense focal dermal lymphocytes and prominent periadnexal lymphoplasmocytic infiltration.

FNAC

Reactive lymphoid hyperplasia.

Bone Marrow Biopsy

Marrow infiltration by atypical malignant cells (blast) with convoluted clefted nuclei, prominent nucleoli and scanty to moderate cytoplasm.

Immunohistochemistry

Marrow. Blast – MPO, HLA-DR_4: positive, CD_4 weakly positive and CD_4 34 Negative.

Skin Biopsy

CD_3 CD_4 positive

Patient was referred to cancer hospital for further management. He was diagnosed as case of acute myeloid leukemia.

> **Tips**
> - In case of unexplained pruritus in an elderly patient, we should never neglect the possibility of maliganacy.

> **Editorial Comments**
> - Before considering rare disease as diagnosis we should consider more common disease first
> - We should rely on histopathology reports along with our clinical findings
> - Internal malignancy can present as many cutaneous manifestation, common being pruritus and erythroderma.

Chapter 22

Rare Case Reports

Nina Madnani

CASE NO. 1

- **Age:** 40 years
- **Sex:** Female

Duration
10 years

History
"White-heads" on both cheeks since last 10 years. The patient had suffered from very mild acne during her teens. She had visited several beauticians, and dermatologists who had done facials and clean-ups/advised various topical agents with no success. She was very disturbed with her skin.

Clinical Examination
Skin surface was uneven with pin-head papules, whose appearance was accentuated on stretching the skin (Fig. 1A). On palpation, these felt firm to hard.

Differential Diagnosis
a. Trichoepitheliomas
b. Closed comedones
c. Cutaneous calcification.

Treatment History

Topical Retinoids
Adapalene (0.1%).

Systemic
Doxycycline 100mg bid
    Patient had no response to the above-listed treatment.
    The surface of each papule was nicked (Fig. 1B) with a 11 no. scalpel blade and the lesion enucleated and removed (Figs 1C and D), as the sequence shown in the images.
    Histopathology was consistent with calcification. The lesions healed with no scarring.

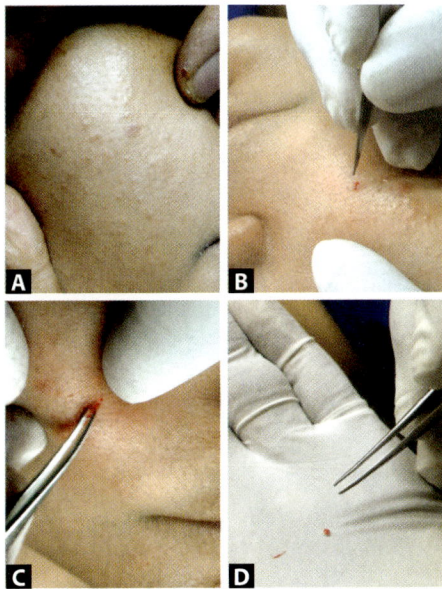

Figs 1A to D: (A) Skin-coloured micropapules on cheek; (B) Skin is stretched and a small incision made over the surface to expose the gritty papule; (C) The papule is separated from surrounding and grasped with a forceps; (D) The removed calcification

> ### Tips
> - Lesions which feel gritty and resemble closed comedones not responsive to treatment, can be cutaneous calcification and should be removed as above.

CASE NO. 2

- **Age:** 55 years
- **Sex:** Female

Duration

5 years

History

Pruritis vulva: 5 years
Dyspareunia: 3 years

Clinical Examination

Loss of normal vulvar anatomy (absent clitoral hood, clitoris, labia minora).

Whitening of the inner surface of labia majora extending backwards to the fourchette and anus, giving a "figure-of-8" configuration (Fig. 2). Surface in some areas with thickening,

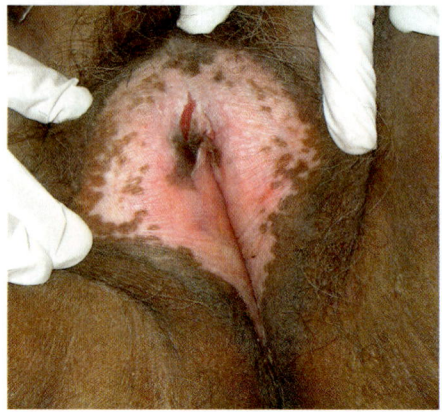

Fig. 2: Vulvar lichen sclerosus showing absent clitoral hood, clitoris, and labia minora

and cigarette paper shiny surface. Satellite atrophic macules suggestive of lichen sclerosus. Vagina spared.

Differential Diagnosis

1. Lichen sclerosus
2. Vitiligo.

Treatment History

Treated with several courses of systemic fluconazole 150 mg weekly, and topic clotrimazole, with no relief.

Patient had no response to the above treatment.
Skin biopsy confirmed the diagnosis of lichen sclerosus.

Treatment Advised

Topical clobetasol propionate application once at night till pruritis abated, and then reduced over several weeks to alternate nights. Patient to be followed up 3 monthly for 1 year, six-monthly, for the next year, and then yearly.

Tips
- Suspect a diagnosis of lichen sclerosus when you see any part of vulvar anatomy missing, with whitening and thickening of the vulvar mucosa, shiny areas with cigarette-paper wrinkling.
- The patients have to be followed up for life.

Editorial Comments
- Common skin lesions like comedones and papules can be presentation of rare condition like cutaneous calcification on HPE.
- Pruritus vulvae should not be ignored and thorough clinical examination should be done with long term follow up.

Chapter 23

Guidelines in Dermatology

PB Haribhakti, Monal Shah, Palak Gandhi

1. Always remember: Diagnosis before treatment.
2. Write short notes when you see a new patient and during follow-ups.
   An attempt at diagnosis should always be made and noted.
   Good record keeping is very helpful in further assessment.
3. Whenever possible and in cases of doubtful diagnosis, always take a biopsy.
   It will give you guidance regarding the line of treatment and builds up patients' confidence in you.
4. Merely prescribing drugs will not help in treatment. Give some time for a brief review of disease, length of treatment required and possible side effects.
5. Avoid topical combination of drugs particularly cortisone with antifungals or cortisone with antibiotics. It not only interferes with the treatment but also tends to give side effects.
   Stretch marks in groins and thighs are mainly due to combination of cortisone with antifungals.
6. Corticosteroids cannot be used indiscriminately. It has given a bad name to dermatologists. A short-term course requires 6–8 weeks of treatment.
   Always taper very slowly, adjuvant steroid sparing drugs like antimetabolites and other drugs reduce relapse rate.
7. OMP is good for children as it has minimal side effects. OMP should not exceed 3–4 months.
   Intradermal injections are good for alopecia areata and some selected cases.
   It should be avoided in chronic lichenified eczema.
   Intramuscular cortisone is good when there are gastric side effects.
8. Cortisone therapy should be given in a proper dosage schedule.
   Diet restrictions are a must while patients are on treatment. Halfhearted doses do not give you any results.

9. Spend a few minutes in explaining your treatment to the patients and see that he/she understands well. Sun exposure should be properly explained when psoralens are used.
10. Photography is very useful. Always take photos of unusual cases, all biopsy patients and for assessment of interesting cases.
11. Avoid unnecessary laboratory investigations. Patients are already burdened with investigations before they come to you. Only relevant investigations are advocated.
12. Use of google to know about the contents of drugs in suspected cases of drug reaction.
    Textbook reference is important in rare and unusual cases.
13. Do not hesitate to take a second opinion or refer to other specialist for related complaints.
14. Do not give false hopes to the patients undergoing cosmetic procedures.
    Counseling is very important to achieve good results.
15. When simple procedure are helpful do not undertake fancy and hi-tech procedures.
16. Prescription should be as short as possible limiting to 4–5 drugs.
    Avoid multivitamins, tonics and other drugs when they are not required.
17. Diet instructions are not required in most situations except for urticaria and related allergic disease. However, our patients are very diet conscious and they feel that their treatment is not complete without diet restrictions, hence, advise simple diet restrictions.

> **Editorial Comments**
> - 'Experience makes man perfect'
> - Senior consultants like our author have eagle's eye developed over a time with their great experience and work.

Orofacial Granulomatosis

CASE NO. 1

- **Age:** 30 years
- **Sex:** Female

Duration of the Disease

2 months

History

History of rash around the mouth after applying some cosmetics, patient was treated by oral and topical cortisone from outside for the same. Then we treated her by oral and topical antibiotics and other supportive treatment.

History of development of new lesions on and off with severe erythema and rash on chest, abdoman, back, arms and legs and dryness around mouth even after starting treatment.

History of spread of lesions to forehead and cheeks even when on treatment.

Clinical Examination

Erythematous rash around the mouth followed by plaques developing on face, also near sides of nose, forehead (Fig. 1).

Differential Diagnosis

a. Sarcoidosis
b. Orofacial granulomatosis
c. Lupus vulgaris
d. Acne rosacea.

Investigations

a. Routine investigations within normal limits
b. Histopathological examination of a skin biopsy revealed nodular tuberculoid granulomatous inflammaion in patchy pattern throughout the submucosa. The granuloma was consisting of lymphocytes, histiocytes and occasional plasma cells. Overlying epidermis had mild spongiosis and slight hyperplasia.

Final Diagnosis

Orofacial granulomatosis.

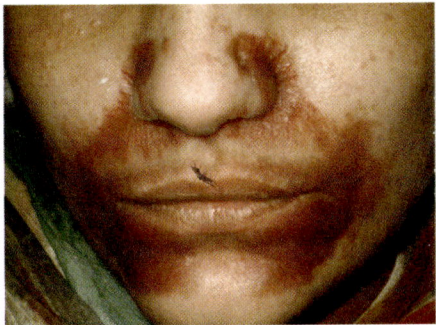

Fig. 1: Perioral erythematous rash

Management

AKT was started. Patient didn't show much improvement after 6 weeks. Then she was given tetracycline 500 mg twice a day, colchicine 0.5 mg twice a day, isoniazid 300 mg and dapsone 100 mg daily for almost a year.

Tips for Managing this Disease

a. Local potent steroids should be avoided on face
b. When the duration of the disease is more than 6 months, biopsy should be taken.

Epidermodysplasia Verruciformis

CASE NO. 2

- **Age:** 25 years
- **Sex:** Male

Duration of the Disease

15 years

History

History of extensive and multiple small to large maculopapular lesions on the face, neck, chest, back, both the forearms, hands and legs:

- History of cryotherapy taken for lesions on arms and chest
- History of similar complaints in younger brother

Clinical Examination

Multiple small guttate lesions on the face, neck, chest, both the forearms and hands.

Some Lesions were Hypopigmented

On arms, legs and back (Fig. 1).

Some Lesions were Hyperpigmented

On face

- Lesions were confluent and pigmented on the face
- Scaling was seen at some places
- No evidence of tumor formation.

Differential Diagnosis
a. Parapsoriasis
b. PLC
c. Psoriasis.

Investigations
a. All routine investigations within normal limits
b. Histopathological examination of a skin biopsy revealed epidermal hyperplasia with slight mammillation on the surface. The epidermis showed vacuolization of cells in spinous and granular layer. Granular layer was thickened. Stratum corneum showed basket weave orthohyperkeratosis with large foci of parakeratosis. Keratinocytes in mid spinous layer showed mild to moderate nuclear pleomorphism.

Final Diagnosis
Epidermodysplasia verruciformis

Tips for Managing this Case
- Treatment is not satisfactory for this condition
- Strict sun avoidance is necessary
- Regular follow-up is necessary to detect malignancy at early stage.

Editorial Comments
- Rare disease presenting in even unusual form is a catch. Skin biopsy in such cases may be rewarding for physicians.

Chapter 24

Leprosy Mimicking as Psoriasis

Rita Vora, Abhishek Pilani, Nilofar Diwan, Nidhi Livani

CASE NO. 1

- **Age:** 76 years
- **Sex:** Male

Duration of Disease

4 years

History

Patient presented to skin OPD with complains of multiple lesions over body since 4 years, pyrexia of unknown origin since 2 months and weight loss since 1 month. He was being treated for psoriasis since 4 years by a homeopathic doctor. There was no complaints of itching, loss of chappals, loss of sensations, ulcers, nasal bleeding. No other comorbid condition was present.

Clinical Examination

Multiple, well- to ill- defined, nonblanchable, nonitchy erythematous plaques with mild scaling over abdomen, back, bilateral upper and lower limbs (Figs 1A and B). There was no loss of eyebrows and no nail changes. B/L ulnar nerves were palpable and nontender. Sensations were normal all over body. There was no motor involvement or trophic changes. Patient had generalized lymphadenopathy.

Differentials

a. Psoriasis
b. Mycosis-fungoides
c. Lepromatous leprosy.

Investigations

All the routine investigations were normal except ESR which was 80 mm.

Chest X-ray was normal. Blood culture did not show any growth.

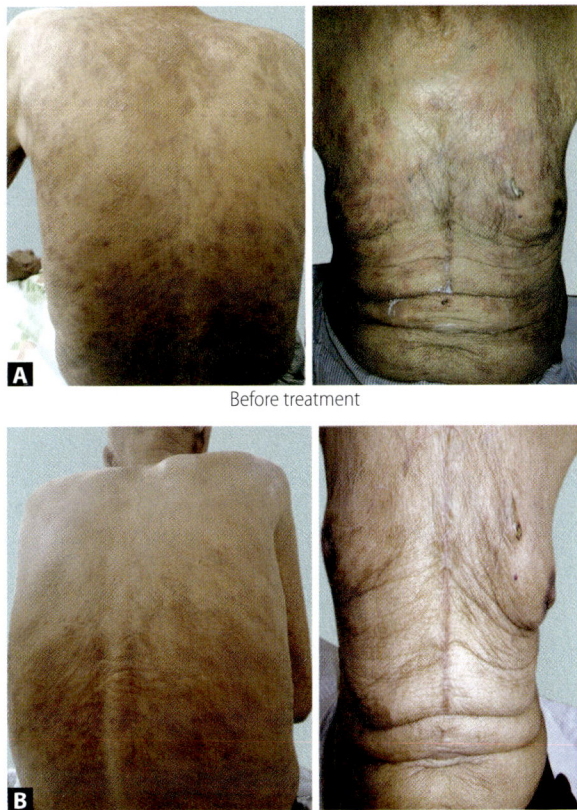

Figs 1A and B: Multiple, erythematous papules and plaques before treatment (A) and response to ALT (B)

USG abdomen and pelvis was normal.

Biopsy revealed thinned-out epidermis, clear grenz zone, poorly formed granuloma containing epithelioid cells, foamy macrophages, lymphocytes and plasma cells. Granuloma involving cutaneous appendages (Figs 2A and B).

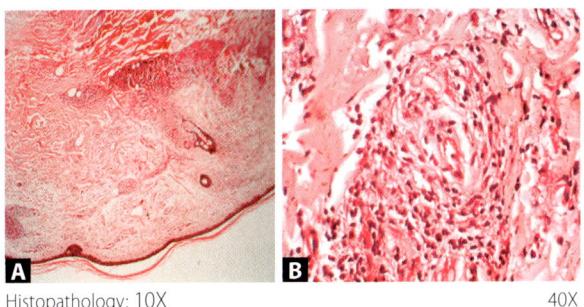

Histopathology: 10X   40X

Figs 2A and B: Granulomatous lesions in dermis (A), lymphohistiocytic granuloma (B)

Following biopsy findings, wade fite staining of biopsy was advised which showed globi of acid-fast bacilli within macrophages (Fig. 3A).

Split-skin smears were positive for acid-fast bacilli (Fig. 3B).

Final Diagnosis

Lepromatous leprosy

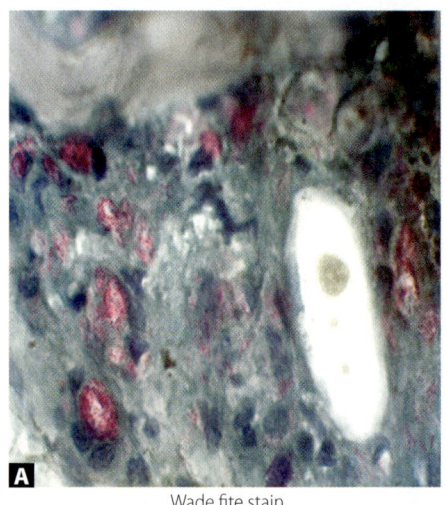

Wade fite stain

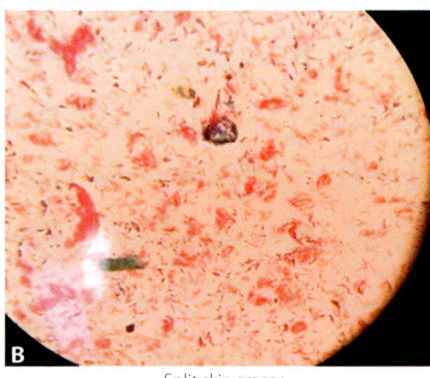

Split skin smear

Figs 3A and B: Special stain on biopsy showing multiple grouped AFB on Wade-fite stain (A). multiple globi on SSS (B)

Management

Antileprosy drugs.

CASE NO. 2

- **Age:** 20 years
- **Sex:** Male

Duration

6 months

History

The patient presented to skin OPD with complains of red raised lesions over body since 6 months.

On Examination

Multiple (>15) well-defined plaques with silvery scales over lower back, abdomen, lower legs were present (Figs 4A and B). He also had swelling over extremities and loss of sensation in a glove and stocking pattern. Nerves were not palpable. Sensations, both temperature and touch were lost in a glove and stocking pattern. No nail changes. Auspitz sign was negative.

Differentials

a. Psoriasis vulgaris
b. Borderline lepromatous leprosy.

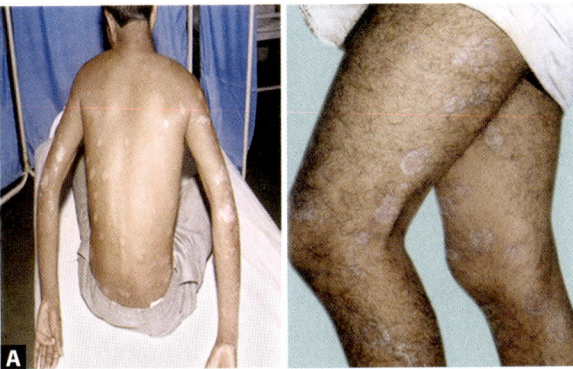
Before treatment

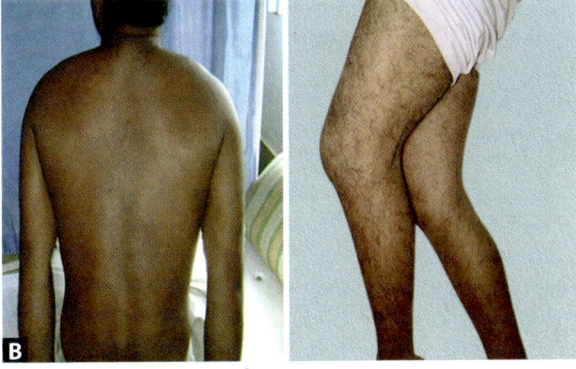
After treatment

Figs 4A and B: Psoriasiform lesions before treatment (A) and after treatment (B)

> ### *Tips*
> - Leprosy is a mutilating and stigmatizing disease. Early diagnosis and therapy is the most important strategy for its control. Clinical diagnosis depends on the history and pathology. If the clinical diagnosis is uncertain, skin biopsy is the gold standard to confirm the diagnosis
> - Leprosy manifests clinically with a bewildering variety of clinical manifestations and may mimic many other dermatological conditions like psoriasis (as seen in our case), mycosis fungoides, urticaria, sarcoidosis, syphilis, etc. Histopathology provides confirmatory information for suspected cases which can be missed in clinical practice and helps in proper classifying
> - There is increasing number of cases with unusual presentation leading to diagnostic dilemma. Only when doctors, other health workers and the population in endemic countries become fully aware of and be able to recognize, the disease in its initial phase, it will be possible for therapy to be instituted at the very beginning. Intervention at such an early stage will avoid the onset of the more serious signs and symptoms, meaning that leprosy will eventually become a less important public health problem
> - Diagnosing leprosy relies on the identification of the typical clinical and histopathological involvement of the skin and nerves. The absence of typical dermatological features greatly decreases clinical diagnostic accuracy and necessitates histological confirmation
> - Even in postleprosy elimination era, the disease continues to be an important health problem. Undetected early cases form a major risk for transmission and disabilities
> - Our cases upholds the importance of histopathology in diagnostic dilemma along with active and sustained surveillance.

Investigations

All the rotine blood and radiological investigations were within normal limits.

Split skin smears were positive for acid-fast bacilli. Biopsy showed clear grenz zone and multiple granulomas in the dermis with foamy macrophages which confirmed the diagnosis of borderline lepromatous leprosy (Figs 5A and B). Patient was started on antileprosy treatment.

Final Diagnosis

Lepromatous leprosy.

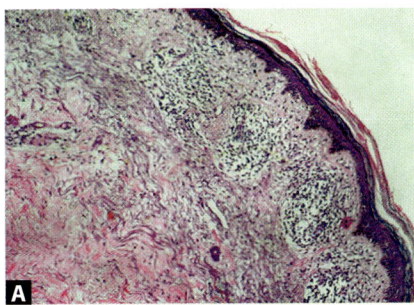
Histopathology: 10X

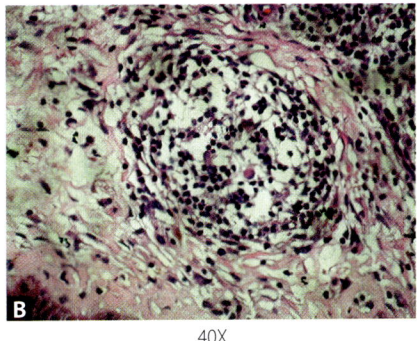
40X

Figs 5A and B: Grenz zone with granulomatous infiltrate (A), well-defined granuloma with foamy histiocytes and giant cells (B)

Management

Antileprosy drugs.

> **Editorial Comments**
>
> - Leprosy is one such disease which mimics many skin conditions and should not be missed by us being a dermatologist.
> - Thorough knowledge and strong clinical suspicion can lead us to correct diagnosis.

Chapter 25

Our Experience with Clinical Dermatology

Ranjan C Raval, Neetisha Agarwal

CASE NO. 1

- **Age:** 40 years
- **Sex:** Male

Duration
Since 4 years

History
C/o generalized red raised lesions all over the body almost daily since last 4 years. During this period patient was admitted for several times for angioedema and extensive urticaria.

Clinical Findings
Generalised erythematous urticarial wheals present almost all over the body.

Investigation
Complete blood count and absolute eosinophil count: Raised
S. IgE: Raised
Allergic skin prick test: Milk protein, jaggery and many more.

Final Diagnosis
Chronic urticaria.

Treatment History
Antihistaminics
- Inj. chlorpheniramine
- Oral loratidine
- Oral cetrizine
- Oral levocetrizine
- Oral fexofenadine.

Corticosteroids
- Oral and injectable

- Injectable histaglobulin
- Oral cyclosporine
- Autologous serum injection intradermal
- Avoidance of milk and milk products
- Patients response to above line of treatment was moderate and temporary
- Again the patient was reviewed and detailed history was taken and that time patient came out with history of taking 'prasad' from temple which was containing milk
- Avoidance of that 'prasad' resulted into complete clearance of the lesions.

CASE NO. 2

- **Age:** 33 years
- **Sex:** Male

Duration

Few days

History and ODP

Generalised maculopapular rash with fever.
Patient had drug history of taking NSAIDs for joint pain.

Patient was admitted and given injectable steroids, antihistamines, antibiotics after which lesions subsided, but every time on tapering steroids flare up of lesions was present.

So patient was investigated for collagen vascular disease, internal malignancy, tuberculosis.

- ANA titer
- Complete blood count
- Peripheral smear
- Urine routine and microscopy
- Liver function test
- Renal function test
- Mantoux test
- Chest X-ray
- Ultrasonography to rule out internal malignancy.

Results

ESR rasied, total count raised, peripheral smear—lymphocytosis.

Skin biopsy was taken and patient was discharged on oral steroids, azathioprine and other supportive medicines.

Patient followed-up with biopsy reports which showed granulomatous infiltration.

Subsequently patient started developing muscular weakness, renal involvement in terms of albuminuria.

Histopathology slide was reviewed and Hansens disease was kept in differentials. Slit skin smears was done which came out to be 6+.

Nerve examination: Infiltrated and thickened ulnar nerve.

Hot and cold sensation: Impaired

Patient was diagnosed with lepromatous leprosy with lepra reaction, hepatitis and renal involvement. Patient was started on antileprosy drugs.

CASE NO. 3

- **Age:** 30 years
- **Sex:** Female

Patient came with complaint of papulonodular discharging lesions in a linear pattern over right leg with palpable lymph nodes.

O/E: Multiple, tender nodules arranged in a linear fashion from heel to mid thigh of right leg. Lesions started as a single painful nodule on heel and then increased in number and size involving whole leg. Lesions were ulcerating and discharging. Edema of the foot with thickened lymph channels along with bilateral hard tender inguinal lymph nodes.

Investigations:

Limb X-ray, KOH and Gram smear done which were both within normal limits.

DD of malignant melanoma and sporotrichosis were kept.

Patient was treated with tablet itraconazole with no response. Thereafter excision biopsy was sent which revealed highly malignant melanocytes invading the dermis, lymphocytic infiltrate and angiogenesis at the base of the lesion.

Diagnosis of Malignant melanoma stage 4 was done. Patient was advised amputation and referred to the oncosurgery department for further management.

CASE NO. 4

- **Age:** 70 years
- **Sex:** Male

Taking antileprotic drugs since 2 years came with complaints of multiple papulonodular lesions over body with few fungating discharging lesions.

No history of tingling numbness, no hot–cold sensation impairment. Slit skin smear negative. Acid-fast bacilli smear negative.

Surgical biopsy was done and diagnosed with Non-Hodgkins lymphoma stage 4 with lymph node and visceral involvement.

Patient was referred to oncology department for further management.

CASE NO. 5

- **Age:** 48 years
- **Sex:** Male

K/c/o acute renal failure on dialysis presented with generalized erythema and papulonodular lesions associated with joint pain and fever.

- Differentials of SLE, leprosy, drug-induced rash were kept
- Complete blood count—polymorphs raised
- Skin biopsy suggestive of polymorphic infiltration
- Patient complained of new crops of lesions with fever spikes.

Treatment

Higher dose of steroid was started and patient responded very well so diagnosis of Sweets syndrome was made.

> **Tips**
> - Common diseases should be always kept in mind first as differential
> - Drug reaction can mimic many common disease and vice versa
> - Always think of Hansen's disease in mind while managing patient with generalized maculopapular rash not responding to systemic steroids
> - Histopathological examination is of utmost importance while diagnosing difficult cases.
> - In any patient history is of utmost importance rather than changing the drug or increasing the dose.

> **Editorial Comments**
> - Benign looking lesions should be considered for malignancy taking into account duration of disease, resistance to treatment and age of the patient.

Chapter 26

Cutaneous Myiasis

Rekha B Solanki

Male, 52-year-old, coming from Africa, came to our skin OPD with chief complaints of painful itchy skin lesions for 8–10 days.

No systemic associations other than diabetes mellitus.

No constitutional symptoms. Vitals were normal. Weight 114 kg.

He gave history of insect coming out of the lesion on squeezing the lesion. Family history of similar complaints in wife.

O/E: Multiple well-defined erythematous lesions with central opening, 7 in number on both thighs, abdomen and back with nonfoul smelling discharge (Figs 1A and B).

D\D: Papular urticaria, parasitophobia

Exploration with forceps and on squeezing the lesion single larva from each lesion was extruded which was live.

Larvae were disposed in turpentine.

Treatment

Topical and systemic antibiotics with ivermectin 200 microgram/kg and anti-inflammatory drugs were given.

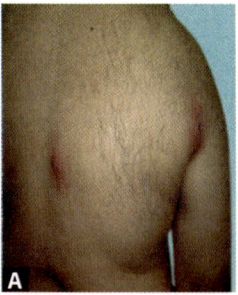 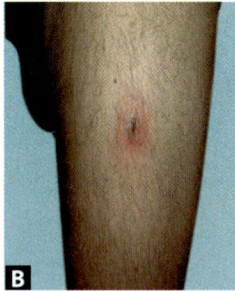

Figs 1A and B: Multiple, erythematous, centrally crusted papulonodular lesions on trunk (A) and leg (B)

Editorial Comments

- Medicine is becoming global now and frequent traveling of people from one to other continent will manifest as changing trends in disease presentations. We must keep ourselves updated with global dermatology!

Chapter 27

Majocchi's Granuloma

Sharmila Patil

CASE NO. 1
- **Age:** 84 years
- **Sex:** Male

Duration of the Disease
More than 6 months

History
Red raised lesions on the left forearm with minimal swelling. History of treatment with multiple antibacterial agents in the past.

Clinical Examination (General and Cutaneous)
Clinically the patient had multiple papules with patches of hypopigmentation and erythema on the flexor of left forearm. Swelling of the forearm was noticed (Fig. 1A).

Differential Diagnosis
a. Angiosarcoma
b. Sarcoid
c. Deep fungal infection.

Investigations
WBC was within normal limit. A skin biopsy was done which was suggestive of nodular granulomatous infiltrate of infective etiology. Biopsy report stated that the upper and mid dermis had diffuse infiltrate of histiocytes and giant cells with interspaced neutrophils and hyperplastic follicular epithelium is seen with the small intraepithelial microabscess. No evidence of malignancy was seen.

Final Diagnosis
Majocchi's granuloma.

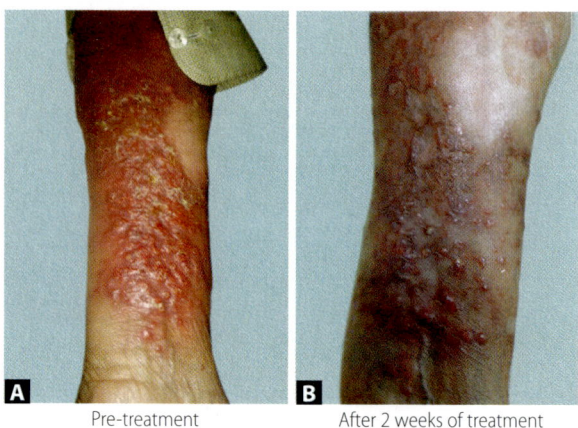
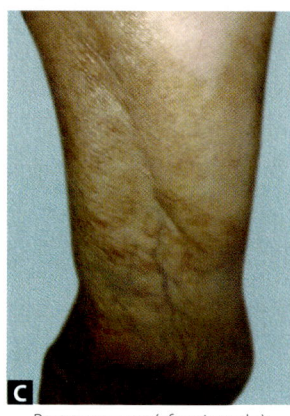

Fig. 1: Lesions pre- and post-treatment

Management

Oral itraconazole 200 mg BD for 3 weeks (Figs 1B and C).

Tips for Managing this Disease

- High clinical suspicion of fungal infection in elderly patients should be kept in mind
- Importance of biopsy and basic fungal scrapping and culture.

Resistant Tinea Corporis Infection

CASE NO. 2

- **Age:** 30 years
- **Sex:** Female

Duration of the Disease
3–4 weeks

History
Multiple reddish itchy raised lesions in the groins, axilla and abdomen. History of treatment with oral terbinafine 250 mg for 2 weeks which did not show any clinical improvement. However, the lesion increased in number and size. History of similar itchy lesions in her 8-year-old son.

Clinical Examination
Multiple erythematous scaly papules coalescing to form plaques with extensive scaling and active border with central clearing over the thigh, groin, abdomen, axilla and infra- mammary area (Fig. 2). Her son had a solitary large, erythematous similar plaque measuring about 6 by 4 cm over the anterior aspect of the left thigh (Fig. 3).

Investigations
KOH mount was done which showed spores and hyphae.

Final Diagnosis
Tinea corporis in family unresponsive to terbinafine (250 mg).

Management
1. Oral terbinafine increased to 500 mg BD
2. Topical clotrimazole BD
3. Counselling done.

Tips for Managing this Disease
- There is an increased incidence of fungal infection not responding to usual oral fungal therapy
- Treatment with 2 different groups of drugs (one topical and the other systemic) should be considered

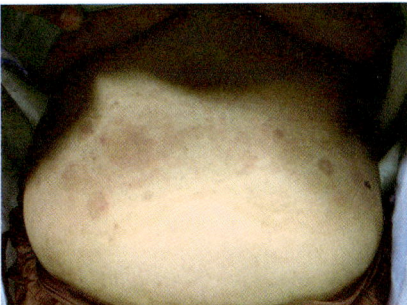

Fig. 2: Scaly erythematous plaque over abdomen seen in the mother

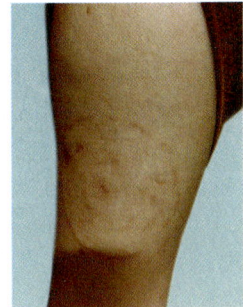

Fig. 3: Circular scaly plaque seen in the 8-year-old son

- Increasing the dose of terbinafine might be helpful
- Oral Itraconazole should be reserved for resistant cases as there might be a rise in the resistant cases in the future.

> **Editorial Comments**
> - Before going to unusual disease common diseases should be kept in mind and histopathology examination can give us the final diagnosis
> - With simpler treatment, disease can be cured nicely if disease is diagnosed properly.
> - Resistant fungus cases are increasing day by day and to treat such cases with close monitoring of liver profile higher doses of terbinafine should be given before shifting to new molecule.

Eczematous Reaction to BCG Vaccination

CASE NO. 3

- **Age:** 3 years
- **Sex:** Female

Duration of the Disease

15 days

History

15 days after the BCG vaccination, oozing eczematous rash at the BCG site as well as forearm and trunk was noticed by mother. No h/o swelling in the axilla. No h/o fever.

Clinical Examination (General and Cutaneous)

4–5 eczematous oval to circular, 2–3 cm sized eczematous patches on the left arm and trunk (Figs 4 and 5).

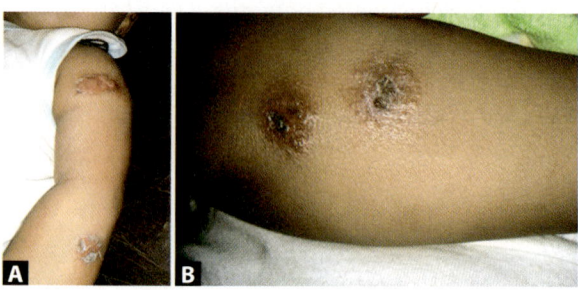

Fig. 4: 15 days post BCG vaccination

Majocchi's Granuloma

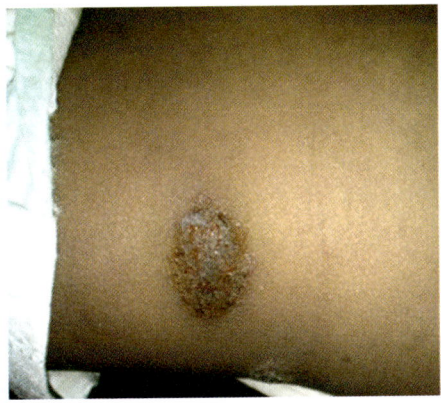

Fig. 5: Subsiding lesion on the trunk

Differential Diagnosis
a. Local reaction to BCG vaccination
b. Lupus Vulgaris
c. Disseminated BCG infection
d. Eczematous reaction to BCG.

Investigations
CBC within normal limits.

Final Diagnosis
Eczematous reaction to BCG vaccination.

Management
Topical fluticasone BD for 15 days.

Tips for Managing this Disease
- Absence of lymph node enlargement in the axilla ruled out postvaccination suppurative lympadenitis which is a common complication with BCG vaccination and requires INH prophylaxis
- Eczematous reactions can be a hypersensitivity to vaccination and can be treated only with topical steroids.

Chapter 28

Interesting Case Reports

Sudhir Pujara

CASE NO. 1

A female aged 24 had been seeing me for recalcitrant pruritic lesions around the mouth. Topical steroids and oral antihistamines would provide temporary relief. She was frustrated and so was I.

Her history was significant for atopic dermatitis for which she had been consulting me periodically ever since she was around 6-year-old.

The lesions consisted of erythema, scaling and crusting. Lesions of atopic dermatitis on usual sites had stopped appearing long ago.

At one follow-up visit she was ebullient and all smiles. I asked her what had replaced her despondence with ecstasy.

Her reply was revealing. She told that her doting mother had been insisting on her to consume eggs since childhood insisting that it was a very nutritious food. Prior to her last follow-up she had been away from home for 10 days where she could not procure eggs. Forced abstinence from eggs solved the mystery of her perioral rash that had ruined her life!

In most cases of atopic dermatitis, allergy to eggs disappears by the age of around 10 and almost in all by the age of 16 years. Peanut allergy may persist longer. In this patient, it had persisted which proved baffling.

Message

Meticulous history taking and some out of the box thinking can be highly rewarding for the patient and the provider.

CASE NO. 2

A male aged 35 had been suffering from recurrent oral ulcers. There was no history of genital/scrotal lesions, symptoms related to eyes or any skin lesions. He had been treated with various vitamins and oral steroids by different doctors but his agony related to discomfort while eating and speaking had no respite.

On examination, he had typical aphthous ulcers. There were no findings to suggest Behcet's disease.

I put him on thalidomide 100mg twice daily and reduced the dose to 50 mg every other day. The whole treatment was stopped after 3 weeks.

Surprisingly, he has remained free from lesions for previous 4 years! Dr. Walter B. Shelley used to say: Lucky doctors get lucky patients!

Comments

My treatment options for recurrent aphthous ulcers (RAU) include:
- A course of tetracycline
- Colchicine: 0.5 mg BD with regular blood counts. Gastrointestinal disturbances are more common. Chronic toxicity includes myelosuppression
- Sucralfate suspension: To be kept in mouth. It is an anti-ulcerant acting by coagulating proteins which form a protective layer making eating comfortable and leading to healing. Can be used 3–4 times daily
- Thalidomide. Constipation and drowsiness (insomnia in some people) are reported to occur but I have not come across such complaints. If long-term or high-dose treatment is required, ask about paresthesias, tingling and numbness, etc. These indicate sensory neuropathy which may be irreversible. Look for sensory nerve action potential (SNAP) changes in NCV study
- Some really stubborn cases may require systemic steroids
- One recent publication has mentioned that even if serum B12 level is within reference range, administration of vitamin B12 may be helpful
- Some patients respond to gluten-free diet.

Lesson

Be optimistic. Be on the lookout for treatment options. Read textbooks and journals and visit the internet.

CASE NO. 3

A male aged 40 presented with recurrent balanoposthitis which had ruined his sexual life. He had received oral and topical antifungals, oral and systemic steroids, metronidazole and several other treatments which had helped only partially and temporarily.

One important piece of history was that a lot of smegma used to collect underneath the foreskin which he used to remove daily. It would come back soon leading to his utter frustration. On examination there was erythema and a lot of smegma.

This history provided me some food for thought. I remembered having read a nice little book written by Dr. John Petitt of Malaysia. Although I had read it several years ago, the lesson that I had learned was pretty much there in my mind. He had proposed that *Mycobacterium smegmatis* which is a commensal can turn pathogenic in some people, producing a lot of smegma and causing irritation and balanoposthitis. I also remembered a simple solution provided by him. 500 mg of clofazimine (from 5 capsules of 100 mg each) was to be mixed with 10 g of vaseline and the ointment was to be applied three times daily for 7–10 days. I got the ointment prepared by a dispensing chemist. Voila! He got permanent relief from this 'irritating' problem (pun intended!).

Subsequently I have treated nearly eight such patients all of whom have been highly grateful to me. What a handsome reward!

The Lesson

Read, read and read. Mark Twain has said: Those who do not read have no advantage over those who cannot read.

> **Editorial Comments**
>
> It can be helpful to search literature often when treating common but recalcitrant skin conditions like balanoposthitis, recurrent oral ulceration as the author has mentioned. As rightly pointed out by author 'out of the box' thinking makes you one step higher clinician.

Chapter 29

Counselling and Peer Discussion: An Additional Intervention in Pemphigus Vulgaris!

Sejal Thakkar

CASE NO. 1

- **Age:** 21 years
- **Sex:** Female

Duration of the Disease

One and a half years

History

She presented with extensive blistering skin lesions associated with oral erosions since one and half year.

She was diagnosed as a case of Pemphigus vulgaris and was treated initially with corticosteroids. Later on Azathioprine and cyclophosphamide were added one by one but she could not tolerate them and finally was put on higher dosages of steroids which could be tapered down for some time, again developing relapse of the lesions.

Clinical Examination

She presented with exacerbation of the lesions along with adverse reactions of steroids in form of Cushing syndrome and extensive striae formation. She was quite frustrated with her condition.

A well-proven case of pemphigus vulgaris with steroid-induced adverse reactions with drug intolerance of other immunosuppressants in a young, college-going student was a challenging task to manage it.

Management

Apart from the management as per the protocol, special counseling sessions were planned for her as she was depressed and frustrated with her condition. She was anxious for her future considering the illness.

During her hospital stay, we had our old case of pemphigus, which was in remission, in our OPD for the follow up. She also had passed through this dreadly situation. Suddenly, it struck my mind to have a conversation between two of them so that this lady can share her experience to the young girl. After taking consent of both the patients, the lady was requested to go to the ward and talk to that girl. By looking to that having remission for so long, the girl could see the hope of being well and have remission. This meeting was followed by various counselling sessions along with the standard management.

Proper explanation with pictorial presentation regarding autoimmunity and nature of her disease regarding relapse and remission was given to her. She was also told about relationship of stress and pemphigus along with role of psychoneuroimmunology.

It made her relaxed and her attitude towards disease was more acceptable.

CASE NO. 2

- **Age:** 30 years
- **Sex:** Female

A known case of pemphigus vulgaris, having off and on relapse since three years was referred from a private practitioner, with extensive lesions and septicemia for hospitalization and management. Patient had lost hope of survival due to extensive, foul-smelling erosions.

At the same time, we had that previous girl of pemphigus in our OPD for the follow-up. She was sent to the ward to talk to that patient and share her experience of remission with very few exacerbating lesions in between since last five years.

This patient was managed as per the standard protocol along with few counseling sessions and over a period of time; she was discharged with good control over her illness.

During the follow-ups, she was much concerned about her postinflammatory pigmentation, weight gain and many more issues.

This gave us an idea to have more interactions amongst the similar patient group and peer communication. The day was fixed in a week for all the pemphigus patients so that they can meet each other and have some tips for trivial issue in day to day life. To initiate, the girl was asked to share her journey like her quality of life during these years, how she graduated, took job in school and now going to marry to a guy of her choice. Other patient shared her experience regarding her gradual weight reduction, control on her salt/sugar diet while on therapy and doing suryanamaskar.

Tips for Managing Group of Pemphigus Patients

It's wonderful to be a part of this peer discussion amongst these patients. One particular day of the week can be fixed for such patients who can come for the follow-up and have interactions amongst them. It will help in dealing with trivial issues of their life and stress reduction. If required, group counselling sessions can also be planned on such days.

Certain tips which I got from my respected teachers and worthy experience:

Psoriatic patients should be advised to comb only hair, not scalp and not to remove the scales keeping in mind the pattern of Koebner's phenomena.

Instruction regarding application/ingestion of the drug should be clubbed with some of his routine task. (e.g. Mind conditioning of application of sunscreen before combing hair may give 20 minutes time for the induction phase.)

Specific and precise instruction for the follow-up, even if the lesions are healed, especially to prevent recurrence must be given (what I say sometimes "if you don't come and continue medicines, it may cause adverse reactions or resistance and if you stop by your own judgment, it may recur as it has been only partially controlled). So, regular follow-up and certain maintenance measures are must to refrain from chronicity of the dermatological disorders.

Chapter 30

An Interesting Case of Necrobiosis Lipoidica Diabeticorum and Trichotillomania: Tips and Tricks

Suresh Joshipura, Deep Joshipura, Vibhakar Vachharajani

CASE NO. 1

- **Age:** 45 years
- **Sex:** Female

Duration of the Disease

2 years

History

Patient had history of lesions over lower legs and shin of tibia since 2 years, which increased gradually. Patient had history of long-standing diabetes mellitus type 2 since 10 years. Treatment was taken earlier from a primary care specialist without any improvement.

Clinical Examination (General and Cutaneous)

Patient had bilaterally asymmetrical atrophic plaques with erythematous or violaceous edge along with telangiectasia over thighs along with a large, 1–2 ulcerative lesion over left shin of tibia (Fig. 1).

Differential Diagnosis

a. Necrobiotic xanthogranuloma
b. Sarcoidosis
c. Lipodermatosclerosis
d. Diabetic dermopathy
e. Sclerosing lipogranuloma.

Investigations

Total count was raised. Although patient was on oral hypoglycemic agents, her fasting and post-prandial blood sugars were raised. Biopsy of the lesions showed thickening of dermis affected by granulomatous inflammation, degeneration of collagen surrounded by palisade of epithelioid histiocytes and sclerosis.

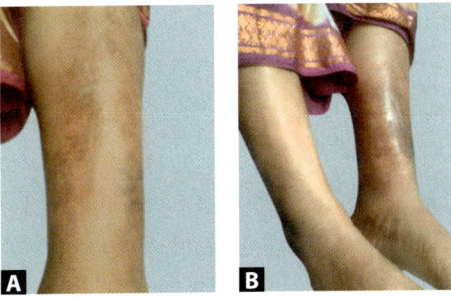

Figs 1A and B: Atrophic, violaceous shiny plaque on shin of tibia

Final Diagnosis

Necrobiosis lipoidica diabeticorum.

Management

Potent topical steroids including clobetasol propionate was given. Oral pentoxifylline 800mg/day was also started. Physician was referred for dose adjustments OHA to control blood sugar levels.

Tips for Diagnosis

Necrobiosis lipoidica diabeticorum is a diagnostic challenge as it always manifest with different morphology. Sharp eyes and strong degree of suspicion to the disease must be present along with good histopathological analysis of the lesion.

Tips for Management

Potent topical steroids must be used, however, care must be taken to avoid systemic corticosteroids since it would worsen diabetes.

Oral pentoxyfylline is often used and often improves the condition by improving local blood circulation. Strangely, control of diabetes has no relation to the progression and healing of this disease.

Proper counseling of patient is mandatory and explaining about the prognosis of the diseases. In long-standing cases, the diseases take a long course to heal due to degenerative changes in collagen due to long-term diabetes.

CASE NO. 2

- **Age:** 5 years
- **Sex:** Male

Duration of the Disease

3 Weeks

History

Patient developed gradually increasing patch of hair loss over frontopariental scalp since 3 weeks. Lesion increased in size with irregular margins. There was a history of habitual pulling of hair from the scalp and habit of thumb sucking. The boy had history of stressful periods in recent time due to schooling.

Clinical Examination (General and Cutaneous) (Figs 2 to 4)

Ill-defined patchy loss of hair over frontoparietal region with presence of short sparse and broken hair. The skin over the scalp appeared normal.

Differential Diagnosis

Alopecia areata.

Investigations

All Investigations including complete blood count were normal.

Dermascopy of patch revealed thinned broken hair attached to the scalp without exclamation mark hair.

Microscopy of the ends of cut hair revealed tapered tips of newly regrowing anagen hair. Hair pull test was negative

Scalp biopsy of the affected areas showed increased number of catagen hair with presence of melanin within follicular canal due to traumatic removal of hair along with absence of perifollicular inflammatory infiltrate.

Final Diagnosis

Trichotillomania

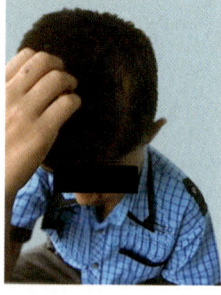

Fig. 2: Child left alone in room, starts plucking hair

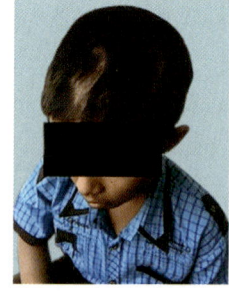

Fig. 3: Child with trichotillomania

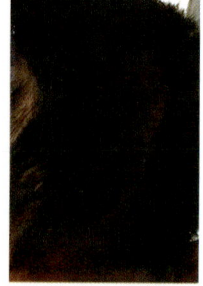

Fig. 4: Hair regrowth post treatment

Management

Counselling of the patient along with their parents was done. Parents were counseled about reducing stressful activities of the child and child was explained about the behavior pattern. Habit reversal training was started and explained to the parents.

Apart from psycho-counseling, topical fluocinolone was given for local application.

Suggested Reading

1. Handfield-Jones S, Jones S, Peachey R. High-dose nicotinamide in the treatment of necrobiosis lipoidica. Br J Dermatol 1988;118:693-6.
2. Lowitt MH, Dover JS. Necrobiosis lipoidica. J Am Acad Dermatol. 1991;25:735-48.
3. Nguyen K, Washenik K, Shupack J. Necrobiosis lipoidica diabeticorum treated with chloroquine. J Am Acad Dermatol. 2002 Feb;46(2 Suppl Case Reports):S34-6.
4. Sawhney M, Tutakne MA, Rajpathak SD, Tiwari VD. Clinical study of diabetic dermoangiopathy. Indian J Dermatol Venereol Leprol. 1990;56:18-21.

Tips

- Generally, in pediatric patients of trichotillomania, the child does not admit pulling of hair
- In such cases, the child is left alone in room and observed for some time. He will habitually start plucking his hair when left alone. By this method we can confirm about his habitual pulling and confirm our diagnosis
- Planning of psychotherapy is most important step
- Counseling of parents, teacher and the child remains a main corner stone of treatment. Habit or behavioral therapy improves the conditions in most pediatric patients.

Editorial Comments

- Psychotherapy plays an important role in treatment and maintenance of certain skin disease like one mentioned by author. It improves prognosis of the disease.
- In uncontrolled diabetes patient when atrophic or erythematous plaques with ulceration are present over shin of tibia then necrobiosis lipoidica diabeticorum should be kept in mind.

Chapter 31

Thorough Clinical Examination is the Key to Diagnosis

YS Marfatia, Ipsa Pandya

CASE NO. 1

- **Age:** 36 years
- **Sex:** Female

Duration of the Disease

4 months

History

Complaint of non-itchy skin lesion around the right eye since 4 months which was associated with occasional pain. There was no history of photoaggravation of skin lesion. There were no constitutional symptoms.

Clinical Examination

A single well-defined nontender erythematous plaque with mild edema was present on the right cheek extending unilaterally up to the right side of the forehead (Fig. 1). Cervical lymph nodes were not palpable. Differential diagnosis considered were leprosy, lupus vulgaris, leishmaniasis, lymphocytoma cutis, lymphocytic infiltration of Jessner.

Sensations were intact over the plaque. Peripheral nerves were not thickened. There was no evidence of facial palsy. This ruled out leprosy clinically.

Oral cavity was not examined hitherto and a look at the oral cavity revealed deep furrows on dorsum of tongue which is characteristic of scrotal tongue. This prompted us to consider Melkersson–Rosenthal syndrome as orofacial swelling and scrotal tongue are characteristic features of the same.

Other differential diagnosis of fissured tongue include Down's syndrome, benign migratory glossitis (geographic tongue), any chronic granulomatous disease, normal population.

Investigations

Hemogram and Routine urine examination were within normal limits, chest X-ray and USG abdomen were normal.

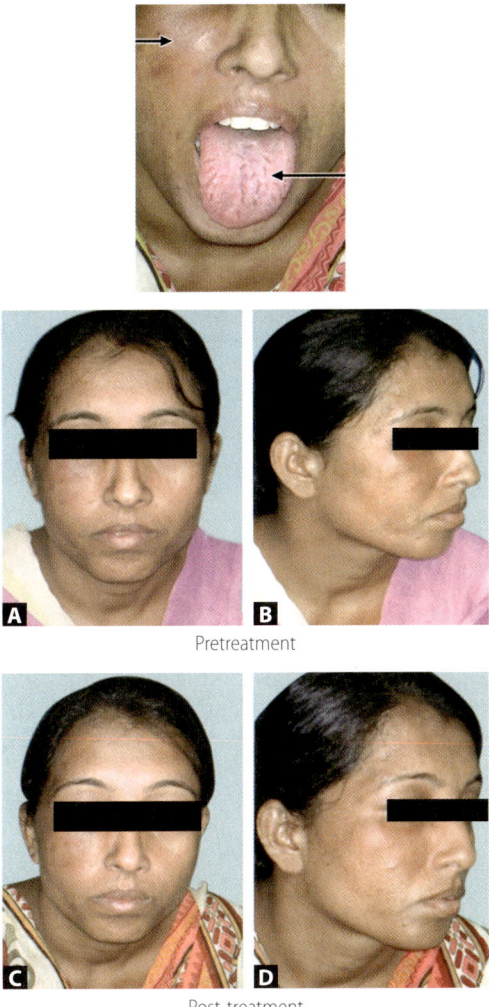

Fig. 1: Shows scrotal tongue and erythematous lesion on cheek

Biopsy was considered but patient was not willing for the same.

Final Diagnosis

Based on the history and clinical examination, Melkersson-Rosenthal Syndrome was considered.

Management

Various modalities of treatment have been tried, which include corticosteroids, doxycycline, clofazimine, metronidazole, azathioprine, dapsone and thalidomide among others.

Tab clofazimine 100 mg twice a day for ten days was given to the patient.

The patient showed marked improvement in terms of reduction in erythema as well as edema which confirmed the diagnosis.

Follow-up care should exclude the development of Crohn's disease and sarcoidosis.

Tips for Managing this Disease

Classical triad of Melkersson-Rosenthal syndrome includes recurrent orofacial swelling, recurrent facial nerve palsy and lingua plicata (scrotal tongue). Since the patient did not have facial palsy, one of the classical features of Melkerrson-Rosenthal syndrome, it can be said that the finding of fissured tongue was significant in clinching the diagnosis. Careful look at the tongue clinched the diagnosis in this case which was further confirmed by prompt response to clofazimine therapy.

The presentation being atypical, thorough clinical examination and a high degree of suspicion is required to make the diagnosis.

> **Editorial Comments**
>
> Atypical presentation of a skin disease may be misguiding sometimes, but detailed clinical examination and wide range of differential diagnosis can make us reach to final diagnosis.

Suggested Reading

1. Medeiros M Jr, Arauio MI, Gumasaes NS, Freitas LA, Silva TM, Carvalhe EM. Therapeutic response to thalidomide in Melkersson-Rosenthal syndrome: A case report. Ann Allergy Asthma Immunol. 2002;88:421-4.
2. Talabi O A. Melkerssons-Rosenthal syndrome: A case report and review of the literature. Niger J Clin 2011;14:477-8.

Chapter 32

Diagnostic and Therapeutic Conundrums in a Case of Pemphigus Vulgaris

Shaurya Rohatgi, Hemangi R Jerajani, Saurabh Jindal, Shylaja Someshwar

CASE NO. 1
- **Age:** 58 years
- **Sex:** Female

Duration of Disease
One and a half years

History
Patient's complaints started one and a half years ago when she developed oral lesions in the form of painful ulcers. Following consultation with an ENT surgeon, the lesions improved but persisted until six months later when itchy, reddish, raised lesions appeared over bilateral limbs and later became generalized. On this occasion, she was treated by a dermatologist for cutaneous and oral lichen planus (LP) with tapering doses of low-dose oral steroids and azathioprine 50 mg per day for one month, following which there was no response. She was shifted to 25 mg per day of cyclosporine, one week following which; she developed reddish lesions and swelling of the lower extremities. Biopsy of the reddish lesions showed signs of vasculitis and in view of drug induced vasculitis cyclosporine was replaced by 7.5 mg per week of methotrexate.

She presented to us with complaints of fluid-filled lesions which appeared first over the lower extremities 20 days back and over a period of 10 days, spread to involve the trunk, upper extremities, face and genitals. The lesions were associated with mild itching and ruptured spontaneously to leave behind raw painful areas. The oral lesions had persisted with varying severity over the past one and a half years, but exacerbated during the present episode. She gave history of weight loss along with decreased appetite over the past one year. No other significant past, personal or family history could be elicited.

Clinical Examination (General and Cutaneous)

Vitals and systemic examination were within normal limit. Cutaneous examination revealed multiple vesicles, bullae and erosions of varying sizes over the face, axillae, upper limbs, abdomen, back, buttocks, gluteal area, genitals and thighs (Figs 1 and 2). Oral cavity and lips (Fig. 2A) showed multiple, tender, irregular erosions and crusting. The scalp and distal parts of the lower limbs were spared. Nikolsky and bulla spread sign were positive. There were no lichenoid lesions at this time.

Differential Diagnosis

Pemphigus vulgaris (PV), paraneoplastic pemphigus (PNP).

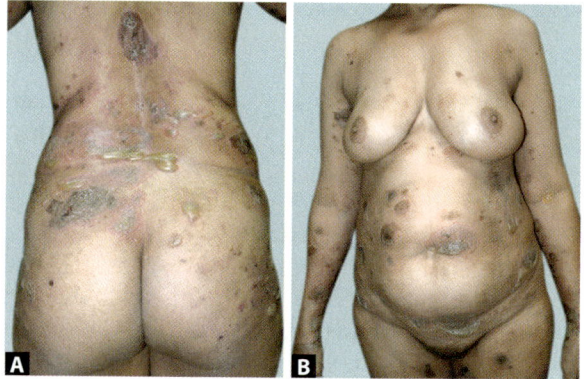

Figs 1A and B: Multiple vesicles, flaccid bullae, erosions with crusting present over the (A) trunk and (B) back

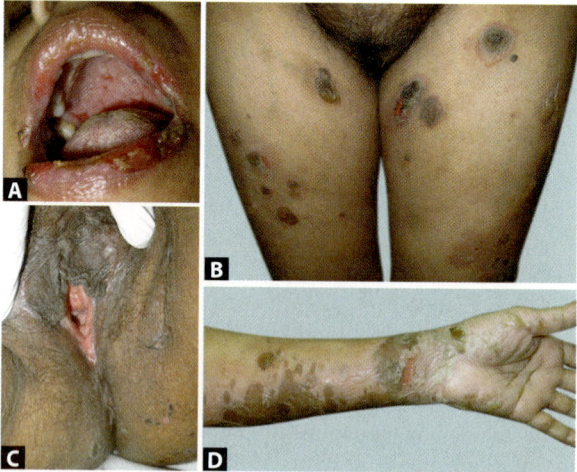

Figs 2A to D: (A) Irregular erosions and crusting present over the lips and hard palate; (B) Few erosions over the vulva, groin and inner aspect of thighs; (C) Erosions, crusting and few bullae on anterior aspect of thighs; (D) Bullae, erosions and crusting over the forearms and hands

Investigations

Hemogram was normal except for leukocytosis. Urine routine and microscopy, blood sugar, renal function tests, stool for occult blood, X-ray chest and USG abdomen and pelvis were normal. HCV, HbsAg and HIV ELISA were negative. Liver function tests were normal to begin with except for low serum proteins. Following treatment with azathioprine, bilirubin levels showed elevation, but liver enzymes remained within normal limits. Histopathology was consistent with features of PV (Figs 3A and B). Direct immunofluorescence (DIF) showed chicken net-like deposition of IgG in intercellular space of the epidermis whereas C3 was seen in a linear deposit at the dermoepidermal junction (DEJ) (Figs 4A and B).

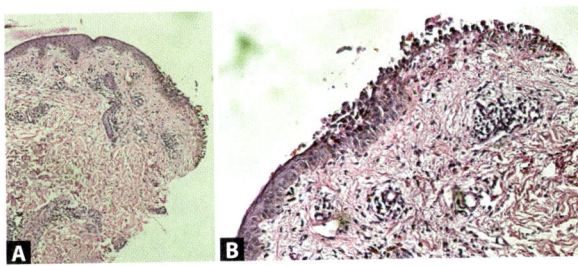

Figs 3A and B: Histopathology: (A) Supra-basal cleft in the epidermis and dermis showing minimal perivascular lymphocytic infiltrate (H and E, x10); (B) Tombstone appearance of the epidermis (H and E, x20)

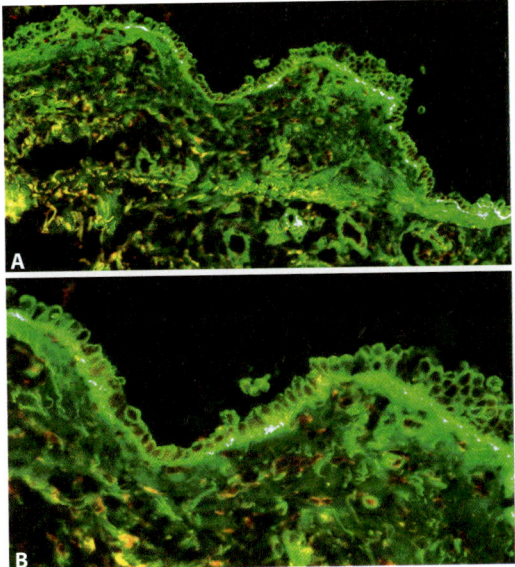

Figs 4A and B: Direct immunofluorescence: (A) Intercellular deposition of IgG along with deposition of C3 in basement membrane zone (x10); (B) Fish-net pattern of IgG deposit in the epidermis and linear patter of C3 deposit in basement membrane zone (x20)

Anti-desmoglein 1 and 3 antibodies levels were positive (142.1 IU/mL and 225.5 IU/mL respectively). Pus culture and sensitivity were done at weekly intervals.

Final Diagnosis

In the absence of any evidence of malignancy, we made a final diagnosis of PV.

Management

Patient's vitals and input-output measurement were strictly monitored. She was started with intravenous antibiotics, fluids and 1 g pulse methylprednisolone (MEP) for 3 days. Oral lesions were managed with potent topical steroid and antiseptic mouthwash. Oral protein and calcium supplements along with protein-rich diet were prescribed. Skin lesions were treated with potassium permanganate dressing followed by topical antibiotic cream. Autoclaved liquid paraffin embedded gauze pieces were used for dressing in addition to plastic sheets on the bed.

Following the MEP pulse, she was maintained with 40 mg per day of oral prednisolone. In addition, we added 100 mg per day azathioprine and this cocktail was continued for 3 weeks after the first-pulse dose. After one month of admission, in view of deteriorating hepatic profile, we decided to start the patient on a modified DCP pulse regimen with 3 days of intravenous therapy followed by inter-pulse oral prednisolone and cyclophosphamide. Few days following the pulse, there was a drastic improvement in the lesions (Figs 5 and 6).

Meanwhile, paraffin gauze pieces were substituted with autoclaved banana leaves for skin lesions along with collagen dressing for few areas, such as buttocks. Protein supplements and high-protein diet failed to improve serum protein levels

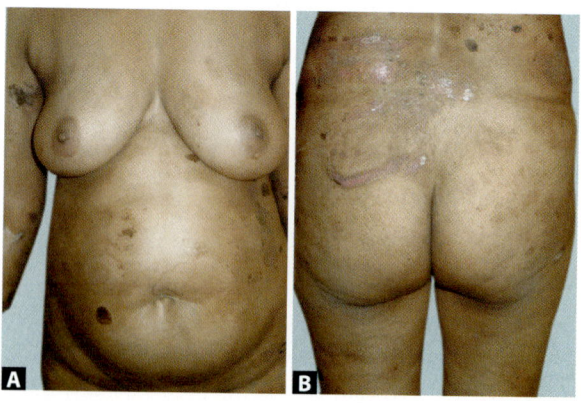

Fig. 5: Healed lesions one-month posttreatment (A) chest and abdomen; (B) back and gluteal area

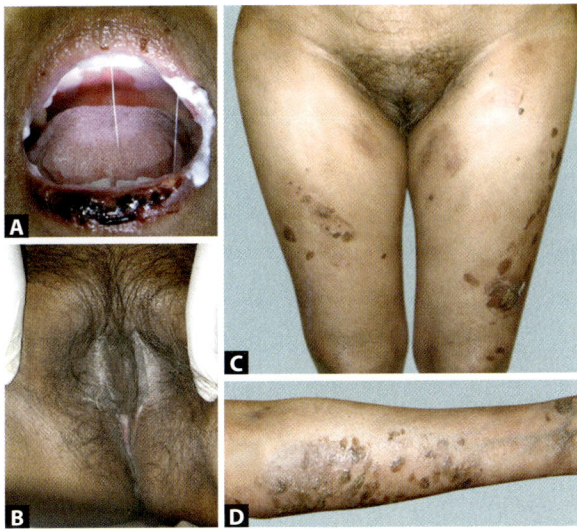

Figs 6A to D: One-month post-treatment: (A) Partial healing in oral cavity; (B) Complete healing over genital area; (C) Complete healing over anterior aspect of thighs; (D) Complete healing over forearms

which kept deteriorating and patient developed pedal edema. Intravenous albumin was administered for three days in an effort to replenish the protein levels. Last but not the least; over this long period of admission, we noticed that the patient showed signs of depression which prompted us to take a psychiatric reference, following which antidepressants were also prescribed.

Diagnostic Tips in this Case

Dermatology primarily being a visual science often presents a diagnostic challenge due to overlapping and ambiguity between clinical presentations. The diagnostic conundrums in this case teach us some important points.

1. The patient first presented with oral erosions for about one and half years but was erroneously diagnosed as oral LP. This is a mistake which is commonly encountered in practise. Oral PV usually presents with irregular erosions which tend to be large in size and are exquisitely painful. Compared to erosive LP, they are more recalcitrant to therapy. In addition, oral erosive LP has a pathognomic reticular pattern, tends to be less painful as compared to oral PV relative to their size. With respect to size also, erosive LP preferentially affects the dorsum and lateral borders of the tongue or the buccal mucosa whereas oral PV affects all areas equally. The surrounding mucosa in erosive LP is often erythematous and glazed, with loss of filiform papillae on the tongue. Oral Nikolsky sign is a

good supportive test to differentiate the two conditions. DIF of oral biopsy sample reliably differentiates the two conditions.
2. Although the biopsy showed features of PV, the diagnostic conundrum at this stage started with the DIF findings which showed deposits both in the epidermis (fish net intraepidermal) and the DEJ (linear C3). In addition, the history of weight loss, lichenoid lesions prior to the development of blisters and recalcitrant oral lesions prompted us to think in the direction of PNP. Even the initial response to standard treatment was poor, which further fuelled our doubts. Although, we could not demonstrate any evidence of malignancy and the patient responded very well to DCP, a high degree of suspicion should always be employed in such ambiguous cases.
3. Antibody levels (anti-desmoglein 1 and 3) would guide in diagnosis and monitoring of therapy as well as deciding the time of termination of therapy. Therefore, it should be done routinely for all cases of PV.

Tips for Managing Disease

The management of a disease like PV seems less complicated in theory which presents multiple choices for drugs and treatment protocols. But applying it in practice while dealing with a recalcitrant, relapsing and resistant case like the one we discussed is an entirely different scenario. We would like to highlight a few therapeutic conundrums we faced while managing this case.
1. Basic nursing care is of utmost importance while dealing with PV. A plastic sheet on the bed prevents the raw areas sticking to the bed sheets. Autoclaved banana leaves smeared with antiseptic used for burn patients can be used for dressing as a nonsticky alternative to gauze pieces. Collagen dressing can be considered for areas prone to nonhealing wounds, such as buttocks and back.
2. Repeated pus culture sensitivity from infected areas can provide guidance to antibiotic selection.
3. Treating for the progressively dwindling levels of serum proteins was an important aspect of management in our case. If protein supplements and high-protein diet do not suffice, albumin infusions can be considered.
4. A one and a half month nonambulatory status dealing with raw oozing wounds, daily dressing and multiple medications with numerous side effects pushed our patient into depression. Therefore, the dermatologist dealing with PV patients should not only manage the disease, but also evaluate any associated psychiatric comorbidity stemming from the debilitating condition. A psychiatric consultation may be beneficial in such circumstances.

Index

Page numbers followed by *f* refer to figure

A

Abdomen, fullness of 63
Acitretin 50
Acne
    excoriee 36
    rosacea 93
Actinic granuloma annulare 6
Adapalene 88
Allergic skin prick test 102
Alopecia
    areata 36, 41, 120
    totalis 7
Amnesia 74
Analgesia, hypnotic 37
Anemia 2, 63, 65
Angioneuritic edema 22
Angiosarcoma 107
Anorexia 63
Antibody 80
Antihistaminics 102
Antileprosy drugs 98, 101
Aphthous ulcers, recurrent
    treatment 113
Ataxia 74
Atopic dermatitis 36
Atypical lymphocytes 29*f*
Azathioprine 123

B

BCG vaccination 110
Bence Jones proteins 8
Biliary syndrome 66
Blaschko-linear
    distribution 61*f*
Blastomyces dermatitidis 11
Blood sugar levels 59
Bone marrow 11
    biopsy 87
Bony lytic lesion 15
Borderline lepromatous
    leprosy 99
Buccal mucosa 30
Bullous pemphigoid,
    prurigo nodularis type 45

C

Cervical lymph node 122
Chlorpheniramine 102
Circular scaly plaque 109*f*
Clitoris 90*f*
Clofazimine 123
Coccidioides immitis 11
Colchicine 113
Complete blood count 26, 59, 60, 102, 103
Corticosteroids 102, 123
Crohn's disease 124
Cryptococcosis 26
Cryptosporidiosis 66
Cushing's syndrome 115
Cutis verticis gyrata 59
Cyclophosphamide 24, 29
Cyclospora 66
Cytoplasmic Birbeck
    granules 16

D

Dapsone 123
Darling's disease 9
Deep fungal infection 107
Demodicidosis 86
Diabetes
    insipidus 16
    mellitus 22
Diabetic dermopathy 118
Diaper dermatitis 15
Diarrhea 66
Down's syndrome 122
Doxycycline 123
Dyshidrotic dermatitis 38
Dyspareunia 89

E

Eczematous reaction 110
Electric dessication
    methods 50
Encephalitis 75

Epidermis, Tombstone
    appearance of 127f
Epidermodysplasia
    verruciformis 94, 95
Epidermotrophism 29
Erectile dysfunction 37
Erythema 52f
    multiforme 31
Erythematous
    atrophic plaques 30, 30f
    lesion 123f
    papular lesions 14f
    papules 1f, 2f, 97f
Erythromelalgia 38
Exophthalmos 13, 16

F

Facial hypermelanosis, diffuse
    management 39
Fever with chills 66
Figure-of 8 configuration 89
Flaccid bullae 126
Fluocionolone acetonide 40
Furuncles 38
Fusidic acid cream 56

G

Gallbladder 64
Geographic tongue 122
Giant cells 101f
Giemsa stain 26
Glossodynia 38
Glycolic acid 61
Granuloma
    annulare 5
    eosinophilic 16
    epithelioid 10
Granulomatous
    disease, chronic 122
    infiltrate 101f
    lesions 97f

H

Hair
    follicles 85f
    loss 41
Hands, dorsa of 1f, 46f
Hand-Schüller-Christian
    disease 16
Hansen's disease 78

Hashimoto-Pritzker disease 16
Hemogram 80
Hepatitis C 80
Herpes
    simplex 38
    zoster 78
Histoplasma capsulatum 9, 11
Histoplasmosis 9, 26
    disseminated 9
HIV
    infection 78
    phobia 37, 38
    screening, types of 78
Hydroquinone 40
Hyperhidrosis 24, 38
Hyperpigmented patches 40f
Hypnosis 35-37
Hypochromic microcytic
    anemia 19
Hypopigmentation 19
Hypothesis 72

I

Ichthyosiform erythroderma,
    congenital 37
Ichthyosis vulgaris 38
Internal malignancy,
    cutaneous manifestation
    of 86

J

Jaundice 66
Jessner's lymphoma 6

K

Keratinocytes 95
Ketoconazole 27
Koebner's phenomena 117

L

Labia minora 90f
Langerhans cell histiocytosis 13,
    15-17
Leishman bodies 27f
Leishmaniasis 122
    cutaneous 26-28
Leprosy 100, 122
    lepromatous 26, 28, 96, 98,
    100

Letterer-Siwe disease 16
Leucocytosis 7
Leukemia 15
Leukocytoclastic vasculitis 29
Lichen planus 24, 37, 41
Lichenoid infiltrate 15*f*
Linear verrucous epidermal
 nevus 60, 62
Lipodermatosclerosis 118
Liver 16, 64
 function test 49, 80, 103, 127
Lower abdominal wall 7
Lung 16
 disease 9
Lupus vulgaris 19, 20, 93, 122
Lusterless hair 42*f*
Lymph node 16
 biopsy 79
 enlargement 111
Lymphocytic leukemia,
 acute 9
Lymphocytoma cutis 6, 122
Lymphohistiocytic
 granuloma 97
 infiltration 27*f*
Lymphoma 82
Lytic bone lesion 16

M

Majocchi's granuloma 107
Malarial parasites 80
Mantoux test 5, 103
Melasma 39
Melkerrson-Rosenthal
 syndrome 122-124
 management 123
Methotrexate toxicity 54, 55
 treatment 56
Methylprednisolone 128
Metronidazole 123
Microsporidia 66
Migratory glossitis, benign 122
Mild oral candidiasis 65, 74
Minimal perivascular
 lymphocytic infiltrate 127*f*
Molluscum contagiosum 50, 51
Mucocutaneous
 leishmaniasis 27
Multiple
 discharging sinuses 19

 erythematous 54, 54*f*
 mildly pruritic skin
  lesions 28
 myeloma 15
 oral erosions 57*f*
 papulonodular lesions 27*f*
 papulovesicular lesions 28*f*
 vesicles 126*f*
Mycetoma 19
Myeloid leukemia, acute 86
Myiasis, cutaneous 106

N

Nail pitting 40
Necrobiosis lipoidica
 diabeticorum 118, 119
 management 119
Necrobiotic
 xanthogranuloma 118
Neurodermatitis 37
Neurofibromatosis 26
Non-itchy skin lesion 122
Nummular dermatitis 38

O

Oil melanosis 39
Oral
 cavity 54*f*
 cetrizine 102
 cyclosporine 103
 fexofenadine 102
 levocetrizine 102
 loratidine 102
 mucosa and tongue,
  infiltration of 27*f*
 Nikolsky sign 129
 steroids 8
 terbinafine 109
Orofacial granulomatosis 92, 93
 management 94
Orthohyperkeratosis 95
Osteomyelitis 19

P

Pain 63
 abdominal 66
Papular tuberculids 86
Papule, needling/pricking of 52*f*
Papulonodular lesions 10*f*, 12, 46, 46*f*, 106*f*

Parakeratosis, large foci of 95
Parapsoriasis 95
Partial aphasia 74
Pemphigus vulgaris 29, 115, 125, 126
    management 128
Perioral erythematous rash 93*f*
Pharyngeal wall, posterior 26
Photodermatitis 6
Photosensitive sarcoidosis 4-6
    management 4
Pituitary gland, compression of 15*f*
Pityrosporum folliculitis 86
Polymorphous light eruption 3
Postherpetic neuralgia 36
Postinflammatory hyperpigmentation 39
Premature ejaculation 37
Progressive multifocal leukoencephalopathy 75
Pruritis vulva 89
Pruritus 38
Psoriasiform lesions 99*f*
Psoriasis 24, 36, 41, 95, 96
    vulgaris 99
Pyrexia of unknown origin 82

R

Recalcitrant warts 50
Renal
    amyloidosis 8
    biopsy 7
    function test 55, 103
Resistant tinea corporis infection 108
Reticuloendothelial system 10
Reticulohistiocytosis 16
Riehl's melanosis 39
Rifampicin 27
Rosacea 37, 38
Rowell's syndrome 30, 31

S

Salicylic acid lotion 56
Sarcoidosis 1-3, 5, 6, 86, 93, 118, 124
    management 2
    plaques of 1
Scalp hair, diffuse thinning of 42*f*

Scaly erythematous plaque 109*f*
Scleredema adultorum 7
Sclerosing lipogranuloma 118
Scrotal tongue 123
Sebaceous nevus 59
Seborrheic dermatitis 15, 86
Sella turcica 15*f*
Serum protein electrophoresis 7
Sexually transmitted diseases 18, 37
Sezary syndrome 55
Skin
    biopsy 2, 10, 14, 27, 87, 103
    disease 6, 12
    lesion 78
Spleen 16
Stratum corneum 95
Stress 36
Subacute cutaneous lupus erythematosus 31
Sucralfate suspension 113
Systemic
    amyloidosis 7
    steroid 77

T

T-cell lymphoma, cutaneous 29
Telogen effluvium 42
Thalidomide 113, 123
Tinea corporis 109
Toxoplasmosis 75
Traumatic nail injury 41
Trichoepitheliomas 88
Trichofolliculoma 83, 84
Trichotillomania 38, 118, 120, 120*f*
Tuberculosis 9, 82
Tubular atrophy 7

U

Urticaria 37
    chronic 22, 38, 102

V

Varicella zoster virus 75
Verruca
    plana 49
    vulgaris 37

Verrucous
    growth 83, 84
    hyperplasia 62
    lesion 83
Vinblastine 16
Vitamin C supplements 40
Vitiligo 38
Vomiting 63, 64
Vulvar lichen sclerosus 90*f*

W

Weight loss 63
Widal test 80

X

Xerosis of skin 47*f*